Recent Results in Cancer Research

Fortschritte der Krebsforschung

Progrès dans les recherches sur le cancer

38

Sponsored by the Swiss League against Cancer

Peo C. Koller

The Role of Chromosomes
in Cancer Biology

With a Foreword by Sir Alexander Haddow

With 42 Figures

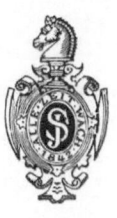

Springer-Verlag Berlin · Heidelberg · New York 1972

Peo C. Koller, Ph. D., D. Sc., Professor Emeritus, University of London. Formerly Professor of Cytogenetics, Chester Beatty Research Institute, Institute of Cancer Research, London

Sir Alexander Haddow, M. D., F. R. S., Professor of Experimental Pathology, Chester Beatty Research Institute, Institute of Cancer Research, London. Former President of Union Internationale Contre le Cancer

Sponsored by Leverhulme Trust

ISBN-13: 978-3-642-80682-7   e-ISBN-13: 978-3-642-80680-3
DOI: 10.1007/978-3-642-80680-3

Peo C. Koller

The Role of Chromosomes in Cancer Biology

With a Foreword by Sir Alexander Haddow

With 42 Figures

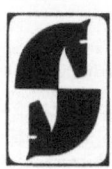

Springer-Verlag New York · Heidelberg · Berlin 1972

PEO C. KOLLER, Ph. D., D. Sc., Professor Emeritus, University of London. Formerly Professor of Cytogenetics, Chester Beatty Research Institute, Institute of Cancer Research, London

SIR ALEXANDER HADDOW, M. D., F. R. S., Professor of Experimental Pathology, Chester Beatty Research Institute, Institute of Cancer Research, London. Former President of Union Internationale Contre le Cancer

Sponsored by Leverhulme Trust

ISBN-13: 978-3-642-80682-7   e-ISBN-13: 978-3-642-80680-3
DOI: 10.1007/978-3-642-80680-3

Peo C. Koller

The Role of Chromosomes in Cancer Biology

With a Foreword by Sir Alexander Haddow

With 42 Figures

1972

William Heinemann Medical Books Ltd., London
Springer-Verlag Berlin · Heidelberg · New York

Peo C. Koller, Ph. D., D. Sc., Professor Emeritus, University of London. Formerly Professor of Cytogenetics, Chester Beatty Research Institute, Institute of Cancer Research, London

Sir Alexander Haddow, M. D., F. R. S., Professor of Experimental Pathology, Chester Beatty Research Institute, Institute of Cancer Research, London. Former President of Union Internationale Contre le Cancer

Sponsored by Leverhulme Trust

ISBN-13: 978-3-642-80682-7   e-ISBN-13: 978-3-642-80680-3
DOI: 10.1007/978-3-642-80680-3

To Karin

Foreword

For many years Professor KOLLER has possessed an international reputation in the fields of cytogenetics and karyology, both in their fundamental aspects and in their relation to the problems of tumour causation, especially to the role of heterochromatin, and few men have made a greater contribution.

The role of the chromosome complex in carcinogenesis has exerted a natural fascination for many decades, but there can be little doubt of the great advances in knowledge and understanding which have accrued of recent years. Although it is probable that the key event in the inception of particular tumours resides in a delicate molecular rearrangement, and is hence undetectable by conventional microscopical methods, nevertheless a large proportion is accompanied by karyotypic variation and relatively gross changes in chromosomal number, order and arrangement, witness the discovery of the Philadelphia chromosome and its consequences. Further, any such changes in the chromosomal apparatus must inevitably be attended by profound repercussions in the cytoplasm with all that this must mean in protein synthesis and cellular behaviour. It would be idle to pretend that any such problems have finally been solved, and they still contain an element of mystery, as can be seen through a quotation from the address given at the Symposium on "Genetics and Cancer", (Houston, 1959) by DARLINGTON, one of the founders of the discipline of Cytogenetics:

"Thus there seems no reason to doubt that variations in chromosome numbers occur in tumours not because they matter more, but because they matter less, than elsewhere ... the cell has become less dependent on nuclear balance than in regular development."

But it is one function of the present work still further to stimulate our comprehension of these remarkable changes. Although mountains of effort have been expended in attempts to decipher the mode of action of the carcinogenic hydrocarbons, amines and other classes of chemical carcinogen—so far with little success or precision—much progress has come of recent years through study of the reactive alkylating carcinogens. At one stage it almost appeared that the tumour nucleus in such cases might bear, as it were, an imprint of the alkylating carcinogen which induced its appearance. Be that as it may, we are now approaching ever more accurate knowledge of highly specific interactions between these substances and chromosomal DNA-molecules, especially the purines, so bringing about alterations in base sequence and other effects upon the chemical integrity of chromosomal DNA, with all the attendant consequences.

The book describes the molecular organization and function of chromosomes, as well as the consequences of chromosomal aberrations in human development. Not the least impact of cytology on medicine has been of a highly practical kind, and thus the book also contains accounts of the cellular features of primary tumours and ascitic fluid, and of the cytological actions of radiation and drugs and discusses their relevance to therapy.

On every ground of timeliness and authority, I recommend it warmly, in the certain hope that it must prove of utmost value, at once to those who are already acquainted with its subject matter and to those who are entering a fascinating field.

May 1972   A. HADDOW

Preface

Transformation of a normal cell to a cancer cell is a biological event; it may be referred to as mutation which occurs either at the level of the gene or chromosome. The latter includes the integration of oncogenic viruses into the host cell's DNA. Whatever the mechanism responsible for neoplastic transformation is, it has eventually to affect the genome of the cell. The physical basis of the cancerous cell behaviour is fixed in the molecular organization of the chromosomes and during mitosis it is transmitted through the chromosomes to descendent generations of cells. Abnormal mitosis is a common phenomenon in tumour tissue and has been recognised to be the main cause of chromosomal irregularities which are characteristic features of cancer cells. Already at the turn of the century the possible role of chromosome changes in the aetiology of cancer was being discussed. The discovery of a chromosomal basis of certain pathological syndromes in man e. g. Down's, Klinefelter's, Turner's syndromes, has shown the consequences of anomalous chromosome constitution, and gave new stimulus for similar investigations in tumours.

During the past decade the study of chromosomal aberrations and their significance in the development and progression of tumours became a rapidly expanding branch of cancer research. It has been demonstrated that most malignant growths are of mosaic composition, containing a variety of cell types distinguishable from normal cells and frequently from each other, by their chromosome patterns. The concept of *selective cellular proliferation* has been derived from information gained by studies on karyotypic variation in the cell population of tumours. Chromosome analyses have already brought a clearer understanding of such dynamic processes as cell competition, selection and adaptation, all of which operate within a cancerous growth and have a role in tumour progression and their response to treatment.

I do not intend to present a comprehensive review of the vast literature which has grown up around this subject, full of many paradoxes, discrepancies and descriptions of unexplained phenomena. My aim is to show the value of the information which has been obtained from such studies by considering the chromosomes of cancer cells as a phenotypic characteristic and not solely as the cell components representing the genotype. I hope that colleagues engaged in diverse aspects of cancer research will find the information in the book of interest and help in their own field of study, and those who wish to enter into tumour cytogenetics may find it a useful introduction.

PEO C. KOLLER

Contents

Chapter 1

Chromosome Structure and Function

The concept that chromosomes are essential constituents of cells is nearly a hundred years old. Genetical studies have demonstrated that chromosomes are the carriers of the genes, which determine the hereditary characteristics of the organism. Molecular genetics has given new insights into chromosomal structure and function, its mechanism of replication, the linear sequence of its repeating units which form the genetic code, and the process by which this code is transcribed into a specific protein structure. The chromosomes and their genes are acknowledged to be the biological basis of human variation in health and disease.

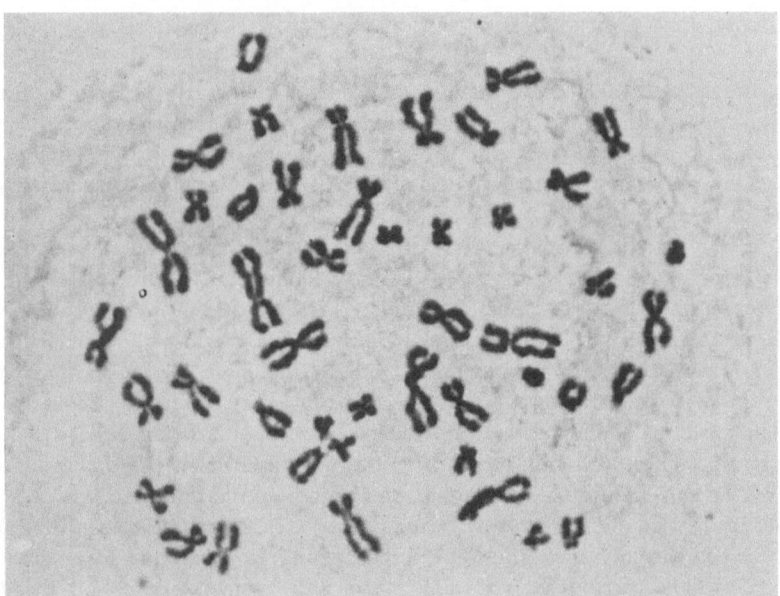

Fig. 1. Metaphase chromosomes of man; each chromosome is composed of two sister chromatids held together at the centromere (By courtesy of Dr. D. T. HUGHES)

The chromosomes can be observed and studied during the metaphase stage of mitosis, when they appear as solid structures, (see Fig. 1).

The core of the chromosome is formed by the double helix of the DNA (deoxyribose nucleic acid) molecule. As well as DNA the chromosomes contain a large amount of basic protein material, which is mostly made up of histones and these very probably act as suppressors in the regulation of gene expression during cellular differentiation. It has been shown that in the organization of the chromosomes, DNA is the material basis of genetic information and provides the basis for genetic diversity, since on removal of DNA by the enzyme DNA-ase, this genetic instruction is lost.

Chromosome shape depends on the position of the *centromere* which represents the "dynamic" centre, and is responsible for chromosome movement during mitosis. the position of the centromere is indicated by a constriction in the chromosome body. According to its position the chromosome can be acrocentric (telocentric), subtelocentric, submetacentric or metacentric, (see Fig. 2).

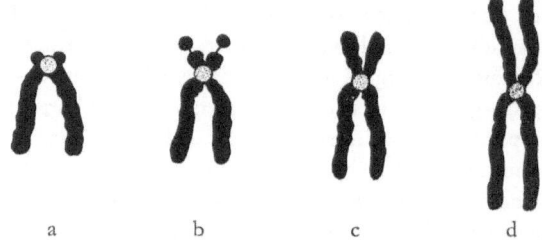

a   b   c   d

Fig. 2. Diagram illustrates various shapes of human chromosomes: a) acrocentric; b) subtelocentric; c) submetacentric; d) metacentric

The short arm of a subtelocentric chromosome is frequently divided into a small distal segment, which is attached with a long secondary constriction to the proximal region of the chromosome arm. The small segment is called the "satellite". The region at the secondary constriction is often associated with the formation of the *nucleolus*.

The number of the chromosomes is characteristic of the species e. g. man has 46, mouse: 40, rat: 42, Syrian hamster: 44, Chinese hamster: 22. Each cell in the body, with the exception of the germ cells, contains the same chromosome number. Within the cells the chromosomes can be arranged in pairs according to their length and shape. In mammalian cells two chromosomes in the male sex do not match; the shorter is the Y and the longer is the X chromosome. The latter has a matching partner in the female, the constitution of *sex chromosomes* being XX, while in the male it is XY. These chromosomes play an important role in the determination of the sex of the new individual. The other chromosomes not connected with sex determination are termed the *autosomes;* in man there are 22 such pairs, and one pair of XY or XX sex chromosomes; the total number being 46 is referred to as the *diploid* number (2N). The gametes or sex cells (sperm and ovum) contain half the diploid number (haploid = N). Cells with abnormal chromosome numbers are referred to as *"aneuploid"* (or heteroploid). This term indicates only the fact that the chromosome constitution of the cell differs from the diploid cell; it is more precise to refer to the chromosome constitution as hypo-diploid, hyper-diploid etc. thus indicating more precisely the relevant deviation from the diploid constitution. The chromosome complement may be present in multiples of the haploid number, thus there are triploid (3N), tetraploid (4N), hexaploid (6N) etc. cells, all of which are referred to as *polyploid* cells.

According to their length and shape human chromosomes have been classified into definite groups. The autosomal chromosome pairs are arranged in decreasing order of size and numbered from one to 22. They are then divided into seven groups represented by the letters A to G. The X is included in group C with chromosomes 6 to 12, while the Y is placed in group G with chromosomes 21 to 22. The arrangement of metaphase chromosomes into pairs is known as the *karyotype;* this term is applied to the systematized array of the chromosomes from a *single cell* prepared either by drawing or by photography (see Fig. 3).

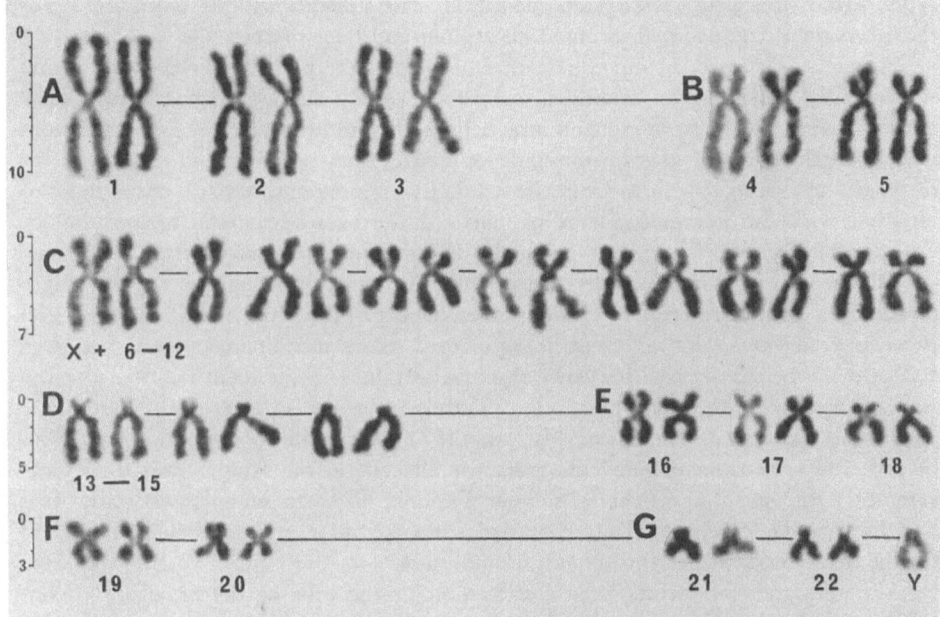

Fig. 3. Karyotype of human chromosomes (male) (By courtesy cf Dr. D. T. HUGHES)

The *idiogram* is a schematic representation of the karyotype, which may be based on measurements of chromosomes in *several cells.*

The characterization of individual chromosomes in the human karyotype is very important, and many other features not only those of length and shape are now being used to distinguish chromosomes within groups. Thus a secondary constriction distinguishes one chromosome in group C; a secondary constriction has frequently been seen in the long arm of no. 16 in group E. Satellites have been detected on all three pairs of group D and on both chromosome pairs of group G. From autoradiography using ³H-thymidine, the sequence of DNA replication in various chromosomes or chromosomes regions was determined; differences in labelling patterns are now used to identify individual chromosomes. Tritiated thymidine labelling during the replication of chromosomes reveals the period and duration of DNA synthesis. It was found that the X and Y chromosomes are late in replication in relation to the other two chromosome pairs of group G; chromosome no. 17 terminates DNA synthesis earlier than no. 18, though both are members of group E.

A new approach to the identification of human chromosomes has been made by
CASPERSSON and his associates (1970). These investigators found that the highly
fluorescent alkylating agent: quinacrine mustard effects discrete, fluorescent labelling
of metaphase chromosomes. Regions fluorescing particularly strongly with quinacrine
mustard have been demonstrated in chromosomes of 3, 13—15 and Y. The presence
in the human chromosomes of specific fluorescent banding patterns as revealed by
quinacrine mustard, is unique and reproducible and thus permits identification of
particular chromosomes (ROWLEY and BODMER, 1971). Computer analysis was applied to the fluorescence patterns of chromosomes within group C and the eight
types within the group have been identified. The method will be most useful for
the detection of translocated chromosome regions and their source.

Staining differences in metaphase chromosomes have been observed visually and
subsequently measured by microdensitometry. Densely staining regions are usually
localised near the centromere and are believed to indicate qualitative alterations
in the organisation of the chromosome structure; they are referred to as heterochromatic to distinguish them from the normally staining euchromatic parts. in combination with the fluorescent banding patterns the heterochromatic regions can be
used as characteristic features of particular chromosomes (CHERNAY et al., 1971).

The two important parameters usually used in karyotype analyses are the length
of the long and short arms of chromosomes. Due to difficulties in the material and
procedure employed by different investigators, these measurements vary between
five and ten percent, which prevents absolute certainty in the identification of part-
ners of homologous chromosome pairs. Through the use of a partially automatic
karyotyping system, GILBERT and MULDAL (1971) were able to compare karyograms
of each cell with the combined idiogram for all cells in the sample, and their measurements showed a significantly smaller variance between homologous pairs than
had hitherto been reported. Their system seems to offer another valuable method
for the characterization of individual chromosomes.

The constancy of chromosome constitution in the cells of the organism corres-
ponds with the stability of the DNA content in the nucleus of body or somatic cells.
Mitosis is the process by which cells keep their chromosome constitution constant,
it ensures that cells derived by this process receive the same number of chromosomes
and the same amount of DNA as contained in the parental cell. Prior to mitosis
the chromosomes and their DNA content replicate. The structure of the DNA molecule was clarified by biochemical and X-ray diffraction analysis The structural organization of DNA is well suited for selfreplication and transcription of genetic
information.

DNA is a large molecule, forming a chain of repeated subunits: the nucleotides,
composed of three parts: base, sugar and phosphoric acid. The bases are of two
types, purines and pyrimidines; the former have a double ring structure, while the
latter consist of a single five-membered ring structure. In the nucleotides of the
DNA molecule there are two pyrimidine bases: cytosine (C) and thymine (T); and
two purine bases: adenine (A) and guanine (G). Many thousand such nucleotides
are joined together through sugar-phosphate linkages and form the polynucleotide
chain of the giant DNA molecule. According to the model of WATSON and CRICK
(1953) the molecule is composed of two polynucleotide chains forming a double
helix in which the base to base attachment represents a series of steps. In this model

one purine base pairs with a pyrimidine base: adenine with thymine (A—T) and guanine with cytosine (G—C) (see Fig. 4).

In the DNA molecule the number of possible variations in the sequence of these four bases is limitless, and it is in the sequence that the genetic information is coded. Segments of varying lengths represent the genes, the primary function of which is the "specification" of protein molecules. Proteins are giant molecules in which many

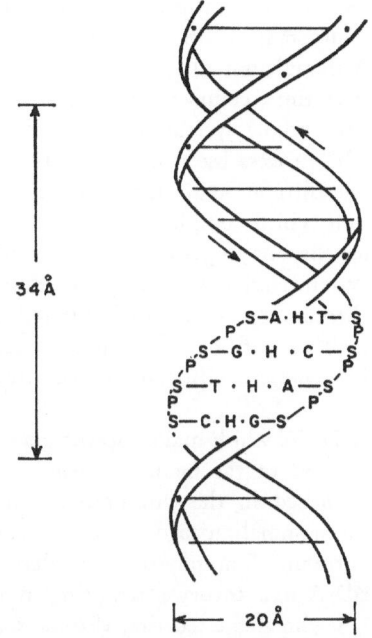

Fig. 4. Watson-Crick model of the DNA molecule: the two sugar-phosphate-sugar chains are held together by hydrogen (H) bonds between their bases, and form a double helix — A: adenine; T: thymine; G: guanine; C: cytosine; S: sugar; P: phosphate group; H: hydrogen bond (After WATSON and CRICK, 1953)

hundreds of amino acids are linked together through peptide bonds, their specific structure and function in cell metabolism depends on the sequence of their amino acid components. Three adjacent nucleotide bases (codon or triplet) in the DNA molecule are required for the selection of a particular amino acid.

The code of the genetic information is embodied in the gene; according to the current concept, the gene is represented by a certain number (600—1500) of purine-pyrimidine bases arranged in a specific linear sequence in the double stranded DNA helix. Recent studies suggest that the chromosome region which is "heterochromatic" is composed of highly repetitive nucleotide sequences. Microbial biochemical genetics provided evidence which showed that in some cases genes coding for amino acids required for one particular protein are situated close together in the chromosome. The function of a gene (or cistron) is that of a template which transcribes the code to a single stranded "messenger" RNA (mRNA-ribose nucleic acid). RNA differs from DNA in having the base uracil (U) substituted for thymine and the sugar ribose in place of deoxyribose. The mRNA molecule leaves the nucleus and in the cytoplasm its base sequence is read by the *ribosome,* on which amino acids are collected. The ribosome is a cytoplasmic subcellular organelle covering the outer surfaces of the three-dimensional network of membranes known as the endoplasmic reticulum. According to the base sequence of the messenger RNA, amino acids are selected and linked together *via* peptide bonds to form polypeptide chains which are then released into the cytoplasm.

The giant DNA molecule with its limitless variation of nucleotide base sequences can store the total genetic information on which the characters and individuality of the organism depends. Although not all genes i. e. all the information coded in DNA, are used at a particular time, cellular metabolism and differentiation are the result of the integration of the whole system *(genome)* as represented by the intact chromosome set. Mitosis is the process by which daughter cells obtain identical genomes. Previous to mitosis the chromosomal DNA replicates, the two parental DNA strands acting as templates on which complementary DNA strands are synthesised. When mistakes occur during the copying of the DNA template, in the process of self-replication, the DNA-repair enzyme corrects the faulty base sequence. It has been observed that if the chromosome structure is altered by physical or chemical agents, or if the genome is either deficient or contains extra chromosome material then this leads to a disturbed genetic equilibrium which affects the behaviour of cell and organism.

Although the structure of DNA which makes up the genetic material of the living organism is now well known, one of the main problems of molecular biology is to find out how the DNA is packed in the chromosomes of higher organisms. The amount of DNA contained in mammalian chromosomes is much larger than is needed to code for all the various proteins. The question is: what is the role of the excess DNA and where is it located? A new theory attempting to answer this question was put forward by CRICK (1971) who suggested that chromosomal DNA falls into two classes: *fibrous*-DNA containing the genes which code for protein, and *globular*-DNA which is located in unpaired regions of the double helix and controls the activity of genes. Just as changes in the genes of fibrous-DNA would result in the impairment of cellular metabolism, so would changes occuring spontaneously or induced in the constituents of globular-DNA. Under this hypothesis malignant behaviour of cells can therefore be attributed to alterations occuring at various levels in the complex organization of the genome.

Summary

Chromosomes are essential constituents of cells; their number and morphology are a characteristic property of the species. The genes are the material basis of heredity and their information is coded in the DNA molecule which forms the backbone of the chromosomes. The structural organization of DNA and its role in protein synthesis have been clarified by molecular biology. The constancy of the chromosome constitution in cells reflects the stability of the DNA content in the nucleus of somatic cells, and this is maintained by the process of mitosis. The chromosomes and their genes are acknowledged to be the biological basis of human variation in health and disease.

Chapter 2

Chromosomal Anomalies as the Cause
of Developmental Disorders

Many instances have been found in plants and animals where both abnormal development and the transmission of hereditary characters were associated with chromosome anomalies. BRIDGES (1916) discovered the presence of an additional chromosome in the genome to be responsible for the anomalous transmission of certain characters in the fruitfly Drosophila. He attributed the abnormal chromosome constitution to be the result of non-disjunction of a particular chromosome during gametogenesis. Similarly in Datura plants, the presence of an extra chromosome in the genome produced new morphological varieties. BLAKESLEE (1922) demonstrated that the different appearance or phenotype of the new varieties depended on which particular chromosome of the genome was "extra". Since that time an impressive amount of information concerning chromosome behaviour in plants and animals has been brought together by cytologists showing that the genetic behaviour of an organism can be inferred and predicted through chromosomal studies.

In view of the fact that many developmental abnormalities in plants and animals have been found to be due to chromosome anomalies, several geneticists considered the possibility that certain aberrations of human development could be associated with chromosome abnormalities. Thus HALDANE (1932) suggested that aberrations in human sex differentiation may have a chromosomal basis; and PETTERSEN and BONNIER (1937) discussed the possibility that chromosome anomalies could explain certain types of human intersex. Similarly PENROSE (1939) considered chromosomal irregularity to be the cause of "mongolism" (Down's syndrome), a view well in advance of the cytological studies which, twenty years later, clarified the chromosomal basis of this condition. In 1937 the present author analysing meiotic division in man observed a dicentric anaphase bridge with acentric fragments, and suggested that this might be due to a structural change (inversion) of a chromosome segment (KOLLER, 1937). But all these suggestions met with opposition from other geneticists who believed that the developmental complexities of a human organism could never be determined by a chromosome set so badly disordered as to be visibly different from the normal.

Studies on the chromosomal basis of inherited or congenital anomalies became possible after 1956 when cytological techniques were improved and the exact number of human chromosomes determined. The misconception prevalent for many years that chromosome abnormalities were unlikely to occur in viable persons was dispelled by the discovery of a large number of such chomosome anomalies. Studies have revealed the association of many congenital abnormalities with particular changes in the chromosome constitution. Human cytogenetics (the study of chromosomes in man) has become of great clinical importance; it is estimated by such studies that in Britain every year nearly 10,000 children are born with chromosome abnormalities, the effects of which range from apparent harmlessness to inevitable death. Every kind of cytogenetic peculiarity previously discovered in plants and animals has now been observed in man. The types of chromosome abnormality that arise naturally or which can be induced experimentally may affect the number or structure of chromosomes, and not infrequently both kinds may be present in the same cell.

1. Numerical Changes

Alterations in the number of chromosomes arise through errors occuring during division, e. g. non-disjunction. lagging of chromosomes, endomitosis, multipolar spindle or failure of spindle formation. When such errors occur during gametogenesis the sperm or ovum will carry an abnormal number of chromosomes and if such gametes become fertilized every cell of the developing individual will have the abnormal chromosome number, provided that the abnormality is viable.

Table 1. Numerical changes and their consequences in man

Chromosome		Syndrome
Number	Constitution	
45	44 + XO	Turner's (female appearance) (1/5000)[a]
47	44 + XXX	Ovarian hyperfunction (mild mental defect) (1/1500)
47	44 + XXY	Klinefelter's syndrome (male appearance) (1/750)
48	44 + XXXX	Mental deficiency
48	44 + XXXY	Klinefelter's syndrome
48	44 + G (21) + XXY	Down's and Klinefelter's S.
49	44 + XXXXY	Mental retardation, skeletal defects, sex anomalies

[a] Incidence of persons in the population born with the syndrome

LEJEUNE et al. (1959) were the first to report an abnormal chromosome number in man. They found 47 chromosomes in the cells of a "mongol" child and suggested the cause to be the presence of an extra chromosome 21 (trisomy-21). Their observations were confirmed within a few months by others, and intensive chromosome studies of many congenital abnormalities were begun. It was soon reported that persons with Klinefelter's syndrome also had a 47 chromosome constitution, the extra chromosome in this case being an X chromosome, (44 + XXY). In Turner's syndrome on the other hand, only 45 chromosomes were found, the missing chromosome being one of the sex chromosomes. The most extensive chromosome alteration was observed in an eight-week old embryo who had a triploid chromosome constitution. Some examples of abnormal chromosome numbers in man and the syndromes they produce are shown in Table 1.

Cytogenetical and clinical studies have shown that the manifestation of a syndrome associated with the same chromosome aberration is not constant or uniform. The effects produced by the excess or loss of particular chromosome can vary; they may be very mild or so severe that they cause death during foetal life.

Table 2 illustrates the complex spectrum of pathological alterations which can be produced by the presence of one additional chromosome in the genome. The wide and variable expression of the syndromes may be attributed to interference by the genes of the extra chromosome with the whole genome. The manifestation of the syndrome can also be influenced by the genetic differences which exist between individuals of the human population.

Table 2. Autosomal trisomy syndromes

Chromosome anomaly	Phenotypic anomalies[a]
D-trisomy (13—15)	Eye defects, deafness, polydactyly, cleft palate, seizures, haemangioma, harelip, anomalous palmar creases, interventricular septal defect, mental retardation
E-trisomy (18)	Failure to thrive, malformed ear, micrognathia, hernia, hypertonicity, defective ossification of sternum, flexion fingers, hip abduction, mental retardation
21-trisomy	Short stature, small round head, protruding fissured tongue, abnormal thyroid function, anomalous dermatoglyphic patterns, immature leukocytes in blood, prevalence to leukaemia in childhood, decreased blood-calcium levels, mental retardation

[a] Compiled from reports of several authors

Trisomy of autosomes is relatively rare and their effects on the individual are so severe that they are usually lethal to the developing embryo as autosomal trisomies not found in life have now been identified in spontaneously aborted foetuses. Theoretically, the genetic imbalance due to the addition of an extra chromosome in the genome can be alleviated by the loss of another chromosome, in which case the chromosome constitution of the cell has been altered but the number of chromosomes remains "normal", though it is referred to as *pseudo-diploid* to distinguish it from the true diploid cell.

2. Structural Changes

Structural alterations are recognised by the new shape and size of chromosomes, or by the irregular pairing behaviour of the homologous chromosomes during gametogenesis; such aberrations do not alter the number of chromosomes in the cell. Most of the reported structural anomalies have been *translocations*, i. e. transfer of a segment from one chromosome to another. Frequently two different chromosomes exchange parts, the phenomenon is referred to as reciprocal translocation or *interchange*. Other structural defects are much less common.

The first case of a structural chromosome anomaly not involving alteration of the chromosome number was described by POLANI and his associates (1960). These investigators found a female "mongol" child who had 46 chromosomes instead of

47, the characteristic number in "mongols". Cytological analysis showed that one of her chromosomes did not conform with the normal pattern, and the anomalous chromosome was interpreted to be the result of reciprocal translocation between chromosome 13 and chromosome 21. The "mongol" girl was trisomic having three chromosome 21's, but the extra chromosome was joined to chromosome 13. Following this report came a similar observation by FRACCARO et al. (1960), in this case the anomalous chromosome was the result of fusion between chromosome 21 and 22, both from group G. These findings are of great importance as they provide the explanation for the familial transmission of Down's syndrome and for the lower than average age of the mothers at the birth of their mongol children in these families, when compared with the other commoner type of trisomic "mongols". In familial "mongolism" the translocations can be found in the "carriers" who are usually the mothers.

The *"Cri du Chat"* syndrome is a condition which is due to structural change in a group B chromosome, it was found that parts of both arms were missing from the chromosome, which usually formed a ring structure. The syndrome was so named because the peculiar sound which the child makes at birth resembles the "cry" of a cat. Individuals with this chromosome anomaly show mental retardation, several minor skeletal abnormalities and heart defects. The very large extra autosome found in association with Waldenström's macroglobulinaemia is assumed to be an *isochromosome*, involving the long arm of chromosome 2 (PATAU, 1961). An isochromosome is the result of misdivision of the centromere, and represents a duplication of chromosome arms. This process has been observed and discussed by the present author (KOLLER, 1938). *Inversion* and *deletion* of chromosome material are other structural anomalies which have been observed in man. A few examples of alterations in chromosome structure are shown in Table 3.

Table 3. Alterations in chromosome structure

Type of change	Chromosomes involved	Syndrome
Translocation	no. 21 — no. 15	Down's syndrome
	no. 22 — no. 13	Mental deficiency, heart disease
	no. 2 — no. 2	Waldenström's macroglobulinemia
	X — X (?)	Amenorrhea
Deletion	Long arm of X	Oligomenorrhea
	Short arm of X	Amenorrhea
	no. 21 (Ph′)	Chronic myeloid leukaemia
Duplication (partial trisomy)	no. 2 (isochromosome)	Waldenström's macroglobulinemia
	X (long arm)	Amenorrhea
	no. 22	Sturge-Weber's syndrome
Inversion	no. 21	Down's syndrome

3. Chromosome Anomalies in the Foetus

The finding of chromosome anomalies in children with congenital syndromes often resulting in early death after birth, suggested the possibility of finding gross chromosomal abnormalities in spontaneously aborted foetuses or still-born infants.

The systematic studies carried out by CARR (1963) showed that chromosomal aberrations are a significant cause of early embryonic death. The interest aroused by CARR's report stimulated further investigations and their results were presented at a conference held in Geneva by the World Health Organization in 1966. The survey covered 450 induced and 800 spontaneous abortions, and revealed that chromosome anomalies are more frequent in spontaneous abortions. The most common type of chromosome anomaly was the addition of an extra chromosome to the genome; the extra chromosome was identified as belonging to the D, E or G group. The relative frequencies of the various chromosome anomalies are shown in Table 4.

Table 4. Chromosome studies in abortuses

Type of abortion		Chromosome Constitution
Spontaneous	Induced	
189	175	normal
72 (27.9)[a]	4 (2.3)[a]	abnormal
261	179	total

[a] Fig. in brackets indicates percentage of total

It seems that at least 25 per cent of all spontaneous abortions are due to chromosome anomalies, in Britain at the present yearly birth rate of 900,000 the annual wastage from chromosome anomalies is estimated to be 25,000 pregnancies.

4. Chromosomal Mosaicism

The chromosome abnormalities described above originate before fertilization, consequently the aberration is carried in the sperm or ovum, and when such gametes are fertilized every cell in the zygote contains the same chromosome anomaly. Chromosomal aberrations however can also occur after fertilization, either during foetal development or in adult life. The most common such anomaly consists of an increase in the number of chromosomes due to non-disjunction of chromosomes during mitosis. As a consequence the individual will have a different chromosome constitution in the cells of various tissues, some will have normal while others will contain the abnormal number. Irregularities arising after fertilization are referred to as "chromosomal mosaicism", a phenomenon which had been well known to occur in plants and animals. The first chromosomal mosaicism were detected by FORD and co-workers (1959) in a patient with Klinefelter's syndrome. Two cell types were found in the bone-marrow; one with 46 and another with 47 chromosomes, the latter constituting the majority of the cells in the sample analysed. The two cell types differed in their sex chromosome constitution, one was XX the other XXY (the characteristic constitution of Klinefelter's syndrome). Instances are also known in which more than two different cell lines were present, and in most cases the abnormal cell lines had altered sex chromosome constitutions. Some examples of sex chromosome mosaicism and the clinical syndromes associated with them are given in Table 5.

Mosaicism involving autosome chromosomes has been observed, but the event is very rare.

The likelihood of detecting chromosome mosaicism depends upon a number of factors: (1) the time of origin of the anomaly in relation to development; (2) the extent of cell migration and (3) the rate of proliferation of the different cell types. Chromosome aberration occuring in *adult* organisms can only be detected when the cell containing the abnormality is proliferative and produces "clones" of cells with the same anomaly. A *clone* has been defined as an asexually produced population of cells, all members of which have been derived from one and the same pro-

Table 5. Sex chromosome mosaics

Chromosome		Clinical condition
Constitution	Number	
XX/XXY	46/47	Klinefelter's syndrome
XX/XO	46/45	Turner's syndrome
XO/XXX	45/47	Turner's syndrome
XO/XYY	45/47	Female in appearance with abnormal gonads
XY/XO/XX	46/45/46	Male in appearance with abnormal gonads
XO/XX/XXX	45/46/47	Variable Turner's syndrome

genitor. As rapidly proliferating cells in adult life are found in the bone-marrow, cytologists naturally chose the haematopoietic tissue in which to look for the possible presence of chromosomally abnormal cells. Most of the chromosome aberrations described previously were detected in the white cells of peripheral blood. By analysing the chromosomes of cultured blood cells from patients with chronic myeloid leukaemia, NOWELL and HUNGERFORD (1960) discovered an abnormally small chromosome in group-G, and they assumed that part of the long arm of this chromosome had been lost. This abnormal chromosome is called the *"Philadelphia chromosome"* and designated as Ph' after the two Philadelphia cytologists who first observed it. The importance of the Ph' chromosome lies in the fact that it is the first chromosome anomaly which is a characteristic feature of a particular malignant condition. Aberrant chromosome constitutions in cells and clones of cells have been observed in the tissues of many human malignancies and represent a special kind of mosaicism in adults. Their unpredictable incidence, lack of consistency and wide spectrum of variability however, make it difficult to evaluate their true significance in relation to the origin, development and behaviour of cancerous growth. The various aspects of chromosome anomalies in tumours will be dealt with in the forthcoming chapters.

Summary

The examples of numerical and structural aberrations in human chromosomes described above show the importance of maintaining an intact genome in the cell. Abnormalities either in the number or structure of chromosomes occuring during gametogenesis, cause developmental disorders of varying severity. Chromosomal mosaicism which occurs in adult life is of special interest in cancer research, as malignant growths have been found to contain cells in which the number and/or structure of chromosomes deviate from the diploid constitution of normal cells. In the light of the findings of human cytogenetics, the study of various chromosome anomalies in tumour cell populations can be expected to yield information which may further enhance our understanding of the very nature of malignancy.

Chapter 3

Mitotic Anomalies in Tumours and Boveri's Theory

The growth of cancerous tissue depends on cell multiplication, and the process by which cancer cells multiply had already drawn the attention of pathologists in the last century. ARNOLD (1879) was the first to describe cell division in human tumours, and cells which he saw containing several nuclei suggested to him that they were produced by "multiple" division of the nucleus. The term "chromosome" was only a year old when KLEBS (1889) described aberrant mitosis in tumour tissue, and noted that in some cells the number of "chromosome bodies" was very large.

The earliest systematic study of cell division in malignant tissue was made by HANSEMANN, who presented the first descriptive cytology of human tumours in a series of papers published between 1890 and 1906. He drew attention to the many

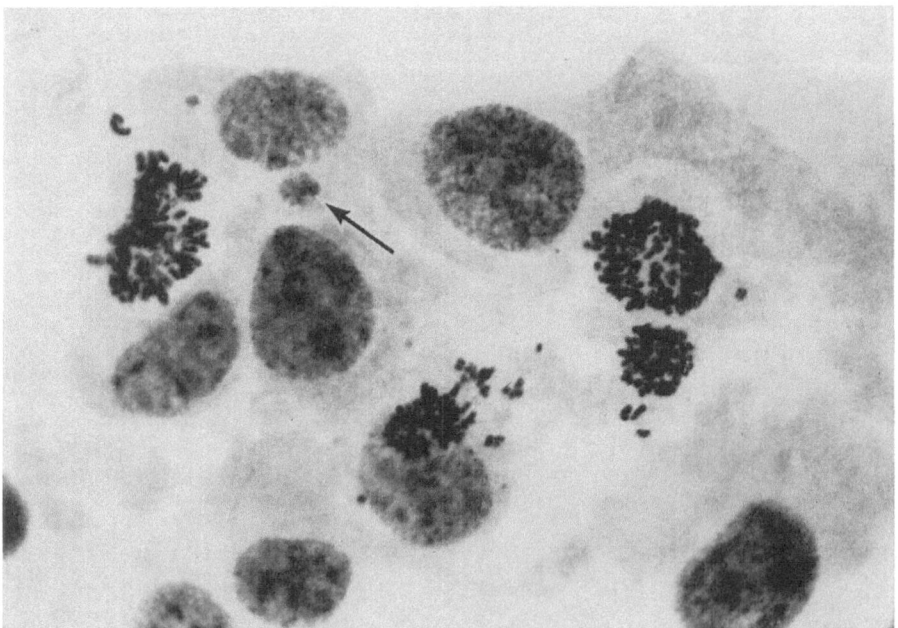

Fig. 5. Dividing cells in carcinoma cervix; showing displacement of chromosomes from the metaphase plate, and different numbers of chromosomes. Arrow indicates a micronucleus, formed by displaced chromosomes; another minute micronucleus nearby in the same cell may represent a chromosome fragment

irregularities occuring in malignant tissue during the process of cell multiplication, and attributed the unusually large or small number of chromosomes seen in dividing cells to abnormal spindle formation resulting in an unequal distribution of chromosomes in the daughter cells (HANSEMANN, 1890) (see Fig. 5).

According to HANSEMANN this phenomenon of abnormal spindle formation could be used as a criterion for diagnosing the malignant nature of the tissue in which they occur. HANSEMANN implied that irregularities during division must result in a disturbed balance between the nucleus and cytoplasm, and suggested that this abnormal balance in the cell is the cause of "neoplasia", a term he used to indicate the deviation of cancerous growth from the normal pattern of differentiated tissues. His view was fully supported by the work of KROMPECHER (1902) who found a very common occurence of multipolar spindles in the dividing cells of 330 human cancers (see Fig. 6).

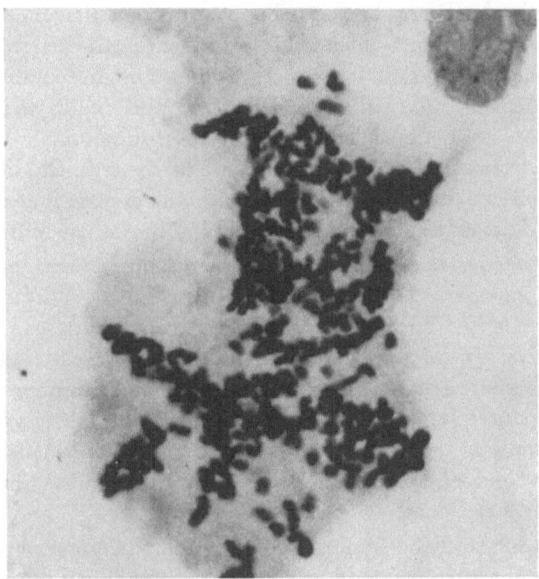

Fig. 6. Metaphase in a dividing cell showing abnormal orientation of the chromosomes due to multipolar mitotic spindle. (Polyploid cell in the ascites of an adenocarcinoma of the ovary)

HANSEMANN's idea concerning the role of a disturbed balance between nucleus and cytoplasm in the cancerous behaviour of cells was further elaborated by BOVERI (1912). He was studying the effect of double fertilization on the cleavage division in the sea urchin egg, and observed spindle abnormalities in the developing larvae similar to those described by Hansemann. As a result of fertilization with two sperms a multipolar spindle was formed, resulting in the irregular distribution of chromosomes between daughter cells. BOVERI referred to this type of cell division as "asymmetrical division". The most important finding was that the abnormal cells thus produced formed themselves into groups lacking the regular arrangement of cells characteristic of normal tissues. BOVERI inferred that the two phenomena: mitotic irregularity and the lack of cellular organization into a differentiated tissue were causally related, and pointed out the similarity between the irregular pattern of cells he observed in the developing sea urchin larvae, and the lack of tissue organization in tumourous growth. These findings led BOVERI to put forward his "Chromosome Theory of Cancer" (1914), according to which malignant growth originates in those somatic cells which have acquired an abnormal chromosome content as a result of "asymmetrical mitosis".

BOVERI'S theory was the first attempt to find a causal relationship between the different phenomena exhibited by malignant growth, and he believed that his theory "may lay a claim to trial if it is able to give a uniform explanation of some of the existing characteristics which never before have been brought into relationship, and if it is able in addition to fit in with other characters". The clinicians and pathololologists of the time being chiefly interested in the identification and classification of cancerous growth, failed to take notice of the theory, although well aware of the various kinds of mitotic aberrations occuring in cancerous tissues. The first cytological evidence in support of BOVERI's theory was provided by the geneticist WINGE (1927). He investigated the Crown-gall "tumour" produced in beet and certain species of tobacco by a bacterium, *(Bacterium tumefaciens)* and found that the majority of cells contained more than the normal number of chromosomes. WINGE (1930) also studied tar-induced tumours in mice, and in spite of the technical difficulties involved in counting mammalian chromosomes, he was able to report that a large proportion of cells had twice the number of chromosomes found in normal cells.

These studies demonstrated that in both plant and animal tumours many cells contain abnormal numbers of chromosomes. According to WINGE, tumour tissue is composed of cells which differ in respect of their chromosome constitution. The concept of *cellular heterogeneity* of tumour tissue is a most valuable idea formulated by WINGE, who visualized the origin and development of tumours as the product of selective processes operating amongst the constituents of a heterogeneous cell population. This concept was a far advanced view of the biological nature of malignant growth which now guides, or should guide, our investigation into the cytogenetic aspect of cancer.

In order to understand the significance of cellular heterogeneity, the mitotic disorders seen in human tumours and observed in experimental tumours of animals should first be described, since they are the mechanism responsible for cellular diversity. Mitotic anomalies in human tumours have been studied by the present author (KOLLER, 1947 a) and are here briefly summarized:

(1) *Stickiness* of chromosomes is one of the most common abnormalities seen in tumour cells, very often resulting in clumping of chromosomes at metaphase. Sticky chromosomes also form "bridges" stretching between the poles of the mitotic spindle, thus preventing the separation of daughter chromosomes (see Fig. 7 a, b, c, d and e).

The configuration resembles paired homologous chromosomes (bivalents) of the meiotic division and because of this close similarity FARMER et al. (1903) made the erroneous inference that "carcinogenesis is a process similar to gametogenesis, abnormally occuring in somatic tissue".

(2) *Non-disjunction* of chromosomes is a failure of the two daughter chromosomes to separate at anaphase. They migrate together to the same pole along the spindle,

and as a result one daughter nucleus contains more and the other less chromosomes than normal. Non-disjunction can be caused by stickiness of chromosomes.

(3) *Lagging* of chromosomes is another anomaly which results in the loss of chromosome material; such chromosomes usually lie outside the mitotic spindle, and at the end of mitosis they may form micronuclei in the cytoplasm (see Fig. 1 and 8).

(4) *Multipolar mitotic spindle* is of common occurence in cells of malignant tissues, and is responsible for the irregular distribution of chromosomes into several

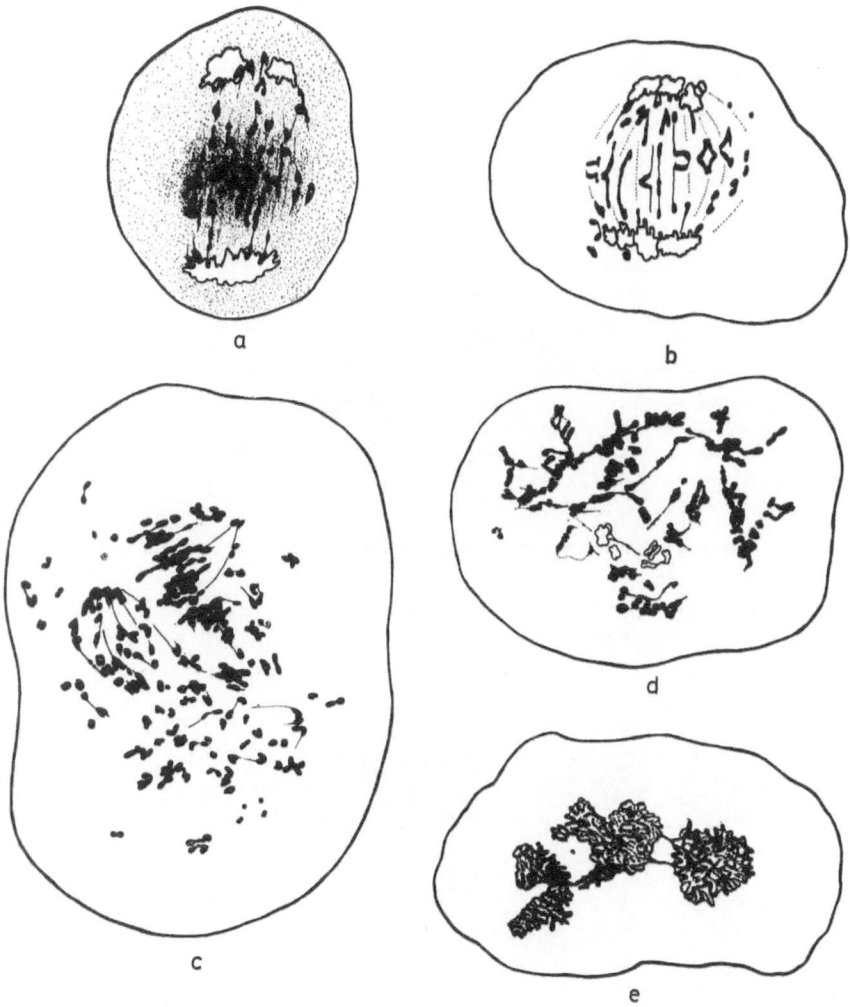

Fig. 7. Camera lucida drawings of mitotic anomalies in tumour cells; a) sticky chromosomes; b) "bivalent configuration" of chromosomes; c) and d) polyploid tumour cells with incomplete multipolar spindles; e) multinucleate cell. (a, b, c: carcinoma cervix; d and e: carcinoma of skin; KOLLER, 1947)

nuclei. Multipolar mitosis is often incomplete, and chromosome bridges hold the various daughter nuclei together. The size of the nuclei varies, indicating that their chromosome content is different (see Fig. 9).

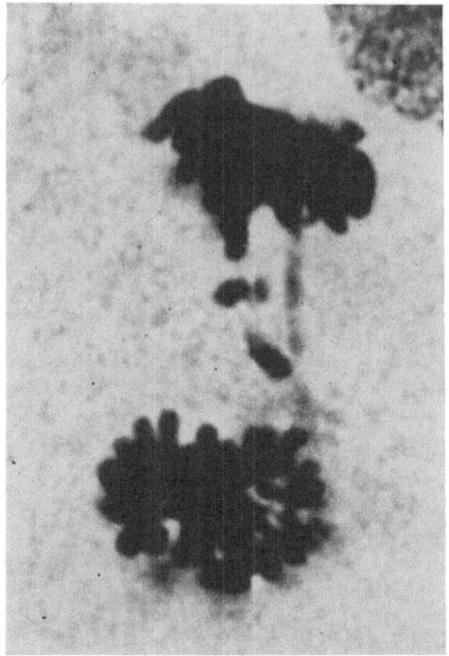

Fig. 8 Lagging chromosomes and "sticky bridge" at telophase (carcinoma of skin)

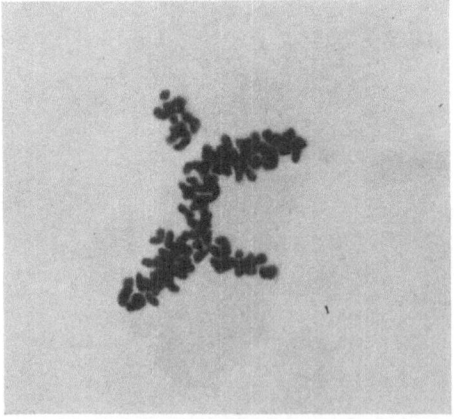

Fig. 9. Abnormal arrangement of chromosomes in metaphase due to multipolar spindle formation; the chromosomes are stained with orcein which does not reveal the mitotic spindle. (Carcinoma of the ovary)

(5) *Binucleate cells* are the result of incomplete mitosis; no cell membrane is formed between daughter cells. At the following mitosis the two nuclei usually divide synchronously, a common equatorial plate is formed where the two sets of chromosomes mix together and the new daughter cells each contain twice the diploid chromosome number. If the process is repeated "giant" cells are formed which may have several hundred chromosomes.

The five mitotic aberrations described above can be attributed to disturbances in the cytoplasmic systems caused by metabolic break-down products which are particularly prevalent in necrotic regions of tumours.

Table 6 shows the frequency of cells with mitotic aberrations in different regions of the same tumour (KOLLER, 1947 a).

Table 6. The frequency of abnormal anaphases (AA) at different regions of a carcinoma

Tumour	Biopsy sites	Periphery		Centre[a]	
		Total no. anaphases	Percentage of AA	Total no. anaphases	Percentage of AA
Carcinoma Cervix	A	151	3.9	51	15.7
	B	97	5.1	48	20.8
	C	241	5.8	93	24.7
	D	119	5.9	131	29.8
Total		608	5.2	323	22.7

[a] Necrotic region

Aberrations affecting the structural integrity of chromosomes also occur in malignant cells; the primary event takes place during chromosomal replication at interphase, but the result can only be observed at the following mitosis.

(6) *Fragmentation* of chromosomes is an example of such an aberration, and is one of the most common anomalies shown by chromosomes of tumour cells. The chromosome fragments are scattered in the cell, and since they lack a centromere fail to move towards the poles at mitosis. The fragments may form *micronuclei* (see Fig. 1) or they may disintegrate in the cytoplasm and will consequently be lost at the next division. The presence of such micronuclei in the cytoplasm is evidence that the nucleus of such cells have lost chromosome material, and the deficient genome may cause the death of the cell.

(7) *Dicentric chromosomes* can be seen at ana- and telophase of mitosis when they form a "bridge" which should be distinguished from the anaphase bridges caused by stickiness of chromosomes. Dicentric chromosomes are the products of breaks in two chromosomes followed by rejoining of the broken parts into a new arrangement. When the two centromeric segments rejoin the result is a chromosome with two centromeres, while the rejoining of the distal segments lacking the centromere

forms the "acentric" fragment. If the region between the two centromeres is very short, the dicentric chromosome can be incorporated into one nucleus in which case it will appear again at the next mitosis. Dicentric chromosomes may prevent the completion of mitosis since the "bridge" formed by such chromosomes holds the daughter nuclei together, resulting in a bizarre shaped nucleus. Very often the dicentric bridge breaks and the broken parts undergo further changes which may be seen at the next mitosis.

(8) *Endoreduplication* of chromosomes occurs during interphase, resulting in the formation of metaphase chromosomes with four sister chromatids. This type of anomaly has been observed mainly in ascites tumours (LEVAN and HAUSCHKA, 1953), it is rarely seen in cells of solid tumours.

The significance of mitotic disorders lies in the fact that (1) they indicate the metabolic instability of tumour cells which are therefore easily affected by environmental factors and (2) they represent the machinery by which cellular heterogeneity is introduced, maintained and increased in tumour tissues. According to WINGE, the growth of a tumour is a dynamic process in which the chromosomal variants of the malignant cell population play a role. Karyotypic analysis (the investigation of chromosome number and form) is the most suitable method for studying the genetic structure of tumours. The introduction of improved cytological techniques and the discovery of free-cell populations of ascites tumours, offered biologists excellent material and methods for investigating the basic principles of somatic cell genetics.

The cytological technique of LA COUR's is an easy and rapid procedure which has been used by cytologists to study chromosome behaviour and to predict the genetical consequences of chromosome aberrations in plants (LA COUR, 1931). The method was adapted by the present author to estimate the effect of X-ray therapy on the cells of human malignancies (KOLLER, 1942). This modified "squash method" of LA COUR's has become the technique now used for the study of human chromosomes by research workers and clinicians.

The first suitable material in which chromosomal differences between cells could be analysed was the free-cell populations of ascites tumours, of which the oldest and best known is the Ehrlich tumour of mouse origin, discovered at the turn of the century by PAUL EHRLICH, the pioneer of experimental cancer research in Germany. This tumour became converted into the present ascites form by LOEWENTHAL and JAHN (1932), fifteen years after the death of EHRLICH. LETTRÉ (1941) made use of this ascites tumour to study the effects of X-rays and anti-mitotic chemicals on its growth rate. In the early 1950's the EHRLICH ascites and its various sublines were intensively investigated by LEVAN and HAUSCHKA (1952). The Yoshida rat sarcoma, another important experimental tumour, was induced by azo-dye in 1943 by Japanese workers, and in the following year the first study of its chromosome constitution was made (YOSHIDA, 1944). These pioneer chromosome studies in ascites tumours have been followed by similar studies in "solid" tumours used in transplantation work, and in primary tumours induced by irradiation, chemical carcinogens and viruses. The early investigators into the chromosome constitution of experimental animal tumours were biologists, chiefly geneticists, whose work opened up an entirely new approach to the study of cellular variability and its significance in the progression of tumours and their response to treatment.

Summary

Abnormal mitoses resulting in altered chromosome constitutions are of common occurence in neoplastic tissues, and can be used as criteria for diagnosing the malignant nature of the tissue. In tumour tissue, cells may have chromosome patterns differing not only from that of normal non-malignant cells, but also between themselves; cellular heterogeneity is a characteristic feature of most malignant cell populations. The significance of mitotic irregularities was recognised by BOVERI (1912) who put forward the concept that chromosomal imbalance is the cause of malignant cell behaviour, and by WINGE (1930) who drew attention to the importance of cellular heterogeneity in neoplastic tissue.

Chapter 4

Malignant Cell Populations and the Stemline Concept

Since the 1950's a great amount of information has been accumulating concerning the cytology of transplanted tumours, many of which were converted into the ascites form. These studies revealed that most experimental tumours were composed of cells differing from normal tissue cells in respect of chromosome number and frequently chromosome structure. The patterns of variation most commonly encountered in the cell populations of tumours are well illustrated by three ascites tumours of mice used by the author. Due to the relatively low chromosome number (2N = 40) and the uniform shape of the chromosomes in mouse cells, murine tumours provide excellent material for cytological analyses.

The first pattern of cellular heterogeneity is represented by C^+-leukaemia in which the greatest proportion of cells have the diploid chromosome number, and as in normal cells the chromosomes are all acrocentrics (see Fig. 10 a).

C^+-leukaemia is a diploid tumour since the cell sample analysed contained only 13 cells out of 55 with either less or more than the normal 40 chromosomes. The ascites lymphoma EL4 reveals the second pattern (see Fig. 10 b).

The cell population is hypo-diploid as the majority of cells contain only 39 chromosomes, which includes a metacentric chromosome. The reduction of chromosome number from 40 to 39 appears to be due to fusion of two acrocentric chromosomes. The cell population of BP8 ascites displays the third pattern of variation in chromosome constitution (see Fig. 10 c).

The largest number of cells (19 per cent) have 69 chromosomes, and the karyotype usually contains one or more metacentric chromosomes; BP8 is therefore a hypo-tetraploid tumour.

The number of chromosomes shown by the highest proportion of cells is the *modal number*, the other cells representing different chromosome variants. The deviation from the modal number might be small involving only one or two chromosomes, e. g. in C^+-leukaemia and EL4 lymphoma, while in others the deviation is large e. g. in BP8. If cells with the modal chromosome number also have *identical* karyotypes indicating that they are descended from a common ancestral cell, they may be considered to be the *stemline* of the tumour. It was suggested by MAKINO (1956) that the cells of the stemline are better adapted towards autonomous growth than the other chromosome variants, and that they are the primary contributors to the growth of tumours. It is very probable that many other chromosome variants are derived from the stemline cells through mitotic anomalies. The frequency of a particular variant indicates its proliferative capacity. In the tumours described above several chromosome variants are represented by a single cell only, which seems to suggest that the abnormal chromosome constitution impairs the capacity of the cell for further multiplication. Such a cell may be considered to be at a "dead end", since though viable it is incapable of division.

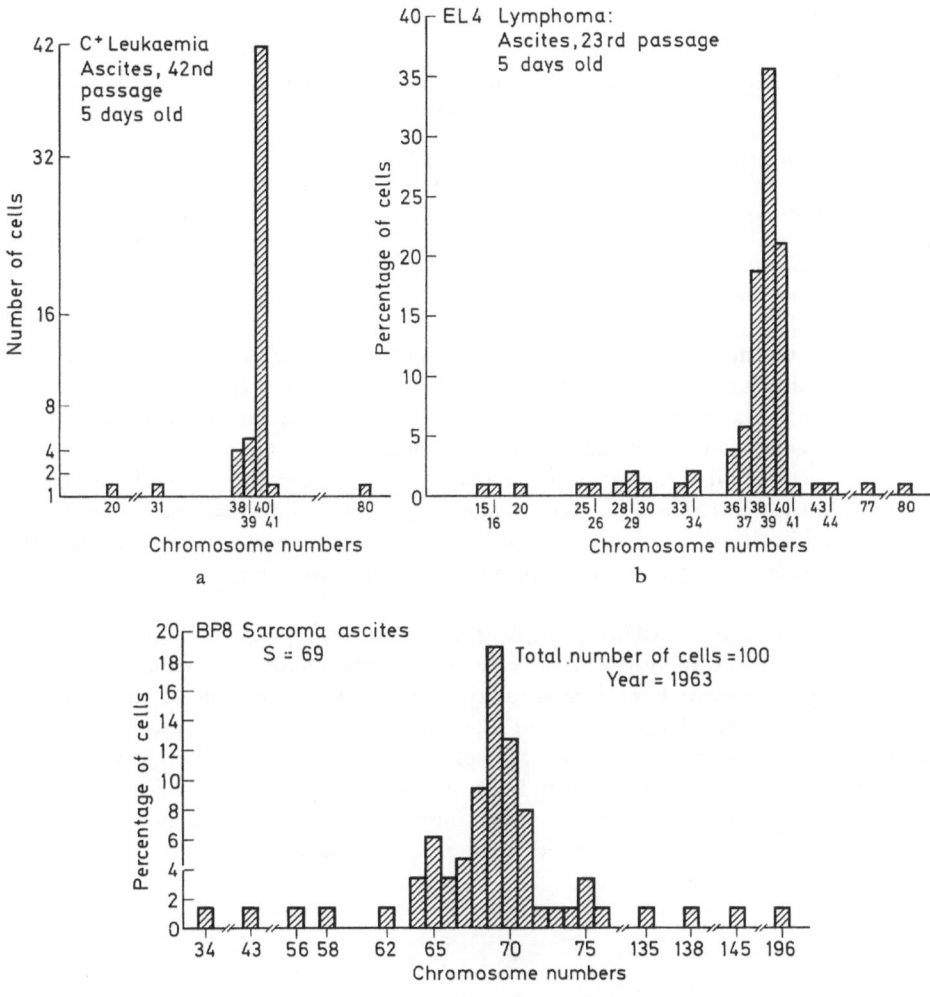

Fig. 10. Histograms showing the frequency of cells with various chromosome numbers in three transplanted mouse ascites tumours: a) C⁺-leukaemia, b) EL4-lymphoma and c) BP8 sarcoma (By courtesy of Dr. A. J. S. Davies)

Structurally altered chromosomes are common in malignant cells, and when the same abnormal chromosome is present in several cells it becomes a *marker chromosome*. Such chromosomes are important since they distinguish tumour cells from normal cells and can also be used to identify clones of cells. Frequently several marker chromosomes are present in the tumour; they may be distributed between different cells or grouped together in the same cell. The combination of marker chromosomes has been studied in the hyper-diploid EHRLICH ascites which contains two easily distinguishable markers: A is a larger than normal acrocentric chromosome with a secondary constriction; B is a metacentric chromosome (BAYREUTHER, 1952). Table 7 shows the distribution of these chromosomes; the highest proportion of cells contained both markers.

Table 7. Frequency of various combination of marker chromosomes in Ehrlich ascites
(After BAYREUTHER, 1952)

Combination of markers	A[a]	AB	B[b]	Others	Nil	Total no. of cells
Frequency in percentage	8.1	61.5	9.7	12.5	8.2	476

[a] A: large acrocentric chromosome with secondary constriction
[b] B: large metacentric chromosome

Marker chromosomes are easy to identify when the structural change results in a new chromosome whose size and shape is grossly different from the chromosomes in the normal karyotype. e. g. a metacentric chromosome in the mouse whose normal karyotype contains only acrocentric chromosomes. *Minutes* are other useful markers; they are very small chromosome fragments with a centromere. Cells of the hyper-diploid Ehrlich ascites contain several minutes, their number varying from two to five. The identification of markers in the human karyotype is difficult since the normal karyotype contains many chromosome types differing both in length and shape.

In tumours maintained by transplantation for many years, the stemline is relatively stable, while in others, especially in recently established malignancies it is variable. Environmental conditions influence the cell composition of tumours, and this is well illustrated by the author's experiments with Yoshida ascites. On subcutaneous injection the free tumour cells of the ascites produce a "solid" tumour. In the peritoneal cavity, besides multiplying in the ascitic fluid, these cells also adhere to the coelomic membranes and develop into "solid" metastatic tumours. The frequencies of the stemline cells in the three localities are shown in Fig. 11.

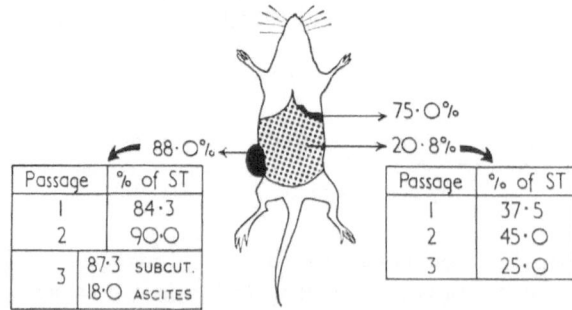

Fig. 11. Diagram showing the fluctuation in the frequencies of stemline cells (ST) in Yoshida sarcoma (CB subline) growing at different sites. The stem cell contains 40 chromosomes, several of which have undergone structural changes

At the subcutaneous site the frequency of stem cells is about four times higher than in the ascitic fluid, and this frequency was maintained during two successive transfers; however, when cells from the subcutaneous site were re-inoculated into the peritoneum, the frequency of stem cells was reduced to that characteristic of the ascites (KOLLER, 1960).

The difference in environmental conditions between laboratories can also affect the cell composition of tumours. An example is provided by a spontaneous mammary adeno-carcinoma: TA3, three derivatives of which were kept by transplantation in the ascites form in three different institutes. The chromosome constitution of the three sub-lines was analysed by LEVAN (1956 a) and is shown in Table 8.

Table 8. Frequency of cells with different chromosome number in three sub-lines of TA3 murine tumour. (After LEVAN, 1956)

Sub-line	Chromosome number																Modal number	Total number of cells
	40	41	42	43 —	64	65	66	67	68	69	70	71	72	73	74+		
TA3/Ha	13	79	7	1	—	—	—	—	—	—	—	—	—	—	—	41	100
TA3/Ki	—	—	—	—	1	3	10.5	17	36	18.5	8	3	2.5	—	0.5	68	200
TA3/KiKo	—	—	—	—	—	—	1	1	4	17	36	19	9	8	5	70	100

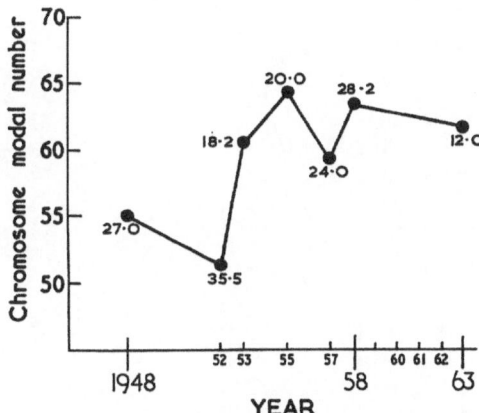

Fig. 12. The variation of the stemline chromosome number in the Walker-256 carcinoma of the rat between 1948 and 1963. The numbers indicate the percentage of stem cells in the cell population

TA3/HA is hyper-diploid having a modal number of 41; the other two sub-lines are hypo-tetraploid with modal number 68 and 70 respectively. The two latter sub-strains have some similar and some different marker chromosomes. The present author determined the modal chromosome number in the Walker-256 carcinoma of the rat which was extensively used in chemotherapy screening investigations. Fig. 12 shows that over a fifteen year time period the modal number varied between 50 and 65 (KOLLER, 1960).

Since Ishibashi's successful transmission of Yoshida sarcoma by one cell inoculation (1950), many tumour clones have been established. The chromosome constitution of several clones of Ehrlich and Krebs-2 ascites tumours of mice were

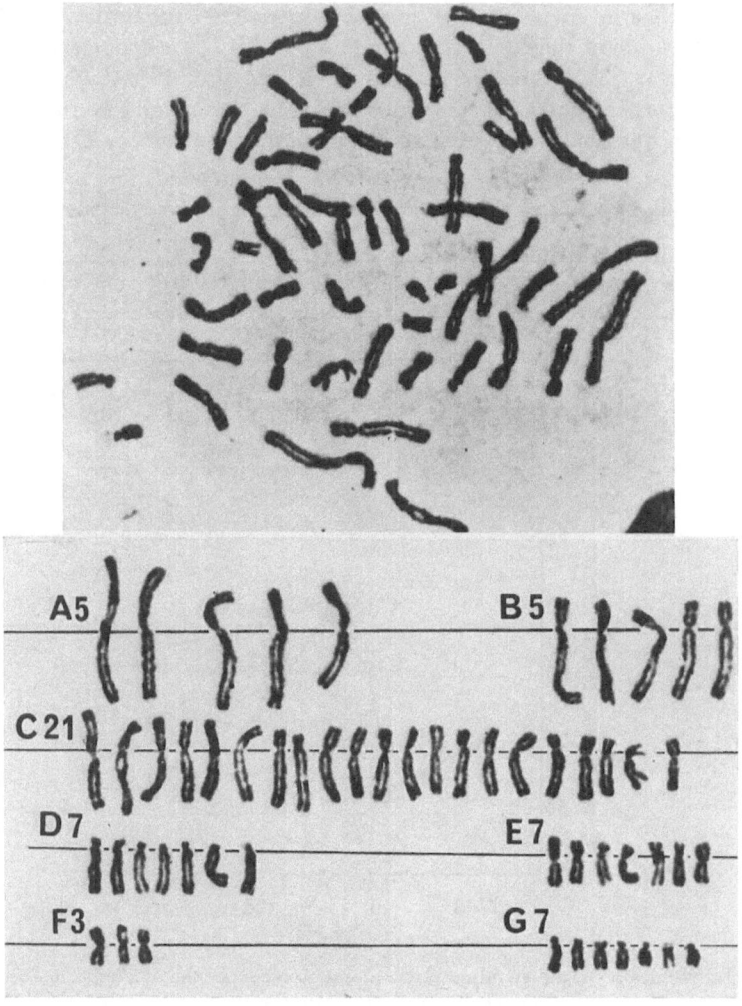

Fig. 13a

Fig. 13. Chromosome constitution and karyotype of two cells in HeLa strain: a) 55 chromosomes, b) 109 chromosomes; in both cells several chromosomes have altered morphology
(By courtesy of Dr. R. J. Belcher)

analysed by Hauschka and Levan (1958), who found a mixed population; the range of variation however was narrower than in the parental tumours. Makino and Kano (1955) made a similar study of single-cell clones of the Hirosaki rat sarcoma. The parental ascites tumour is characterized by the presence of a metacentric chromosome.

The frequency of cells containing different numbers of the metacentric marker was determined in the 22nd and 73rd passage, and the data are shown in Table 9.

While in the 22nd passage cells with four markers were the most common, the 73rd passage contained a higher frequency of cells with three marker chromosomes.

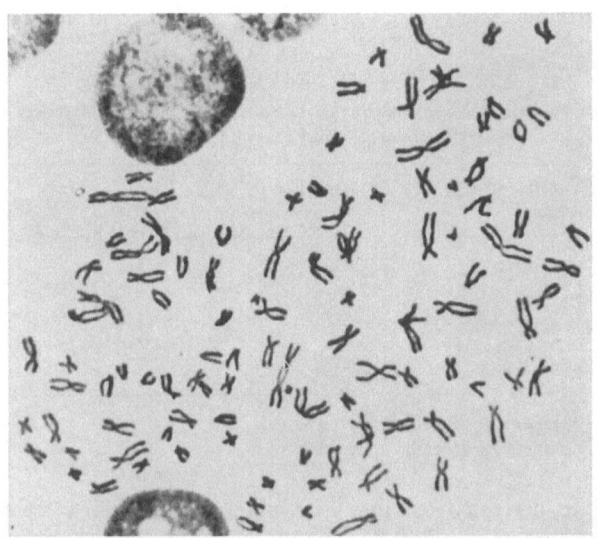

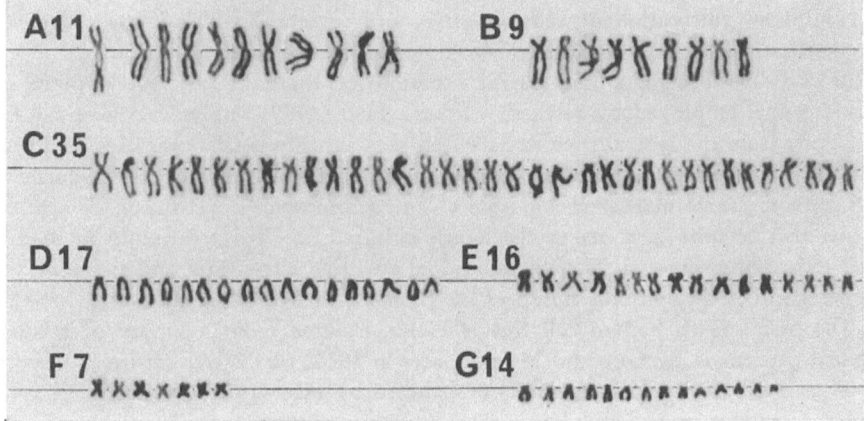

Fig. 13b

From the mixed cell population of the 73rd passage four single-cell clones were established. In two clones the predominant cell type had two markers, in the other two it had three; this finding reflects the most common cell types in the mixed population of the parental tumour. Many clones of tumours have been found which contain chromosome types not present in the parental tumour. The appearance of new marker chromosomes indicates that structural rearrangements have occured after the clones were established.

The cell populations of most experimental tumours undergo further changes during their propagation by transplantation, and these changes may be responsible for the inconsistent results obtained in experiments in which the tumours were used. It is now well documented that tumour sub-lines derived from a common ancestral tumour often have chromosome characteristics different from the parental tumour. Furthermore, tumours believed to be identical since they have the same name, but maintained in different laboratories were found to have chromosomally different cell populations.

Table 9. Frequency of cells with marker chromosomes in Hirosaki sarcoma of the rat
(After MAKINO and KANO, 1955)

Number of markers in cells	Passage 22nd[a]	Passage 73rd[b]
1	2.9	5.7
2	17.4	40.3
3	20.3	44.0
4	50.7	10.0
5	8.7	nil

[a] percent of 85 cells analysed
[b] percent of 76 cells analysed

Cell populations derived from tumour explants cultured *in vitro* have also been the subject of chromosomal studies. EARLE (1943) was the first to adapt the technique of continuous cultivation of cells *in vitro*, and to establish the L-strain from the subcutaneous tissue of a mouse which had been treated with a carcinogen. The L-strain of EARLE became a very useful experimental material and several of its sub-lines are now employed by research workers. HSU (1959) analysed twelve sub-lines of a clone from the L-strain which had been kept in different laboratories, and found that they differed in respect of the number of chromosomes and the frequency of cells with the same marker chromosomes. The chromosome constitution of nine substrains of a lympho-sarcoma of the mouse cultured *in vitro* was found to be different, each subline having its own individual stemline karyotype and range of variation regarding chromosome number (DE BRUYN and HANSEN-MELANDER, 1958).

The best known human cell line is HeLa, isolated from a biopsy of a human cervical carcinoma by GEY and his associates in 1952. HeLa was grown *in vitro* for three years before its chromosomes were studied by HSU (1954 a) who found a very wide spectrum of variation in chromosome number, ranging from 50 to several hundreds, and reported the modal number to be 83. The chromosomal constitution of secondary clones of HeLa were analysed by CHU and GILES (1958) who observed different numerical and structural changes in the various clones, and differences in the frequency of cells with the modal chromosome number. Great variation was also found in the frequency of mitotic abnormalities; in one clone it was 3.6 per cent and in another 16.7 per cent. These investigators reported that while the clones were under observation dicentric chromosomes appeared in several cells.

Fig. 13 a and b show the chromosome constitution in two cells of the HeLa strain maintained in our laboratory; one has 55 and the other 109 chromosomes. Four human tumour strains, H.S1, H.EP1, 2 and 3 were analysed three years after the strains were established by Dr. H. TOOLAN in 1953; two were hyper-diploid, one was hypo-triploid and the fourth was tetraploid (LEVAN, 1956 b).

The most interesting discovery however, was the finding that cell populations derived from *non-malignant* tissues and cultured *in vitro* also showed extensive alterations in chromosome constitution. The alterations occur gradually and may result in the complete disappearance of diploid cells with normal karyotypes. This phenomenon is referred to as "heteroploid transformation" and was first reported by HSU and MOORHEAD (1957). These workers cultured a tissue explant obtained from the synovial lining of a man, and found that up to the fifth passage most of the cells were diploid with 46 chromosomes. In the eighth sub-culture only cells containing more than 46 were seen and some cells had over a hundred chromosomes.

During the past ten years several human cell strains were established; under strict culturing conditions some retained the diploid or near diploid pattern, but most of them developed grossly altered chromosome constitutions, the modal number commonly lying between 60 and 70. The pattern of chromosomal changes occuring *in vitro* has been studied by HSU (1960), according to whom the first significant change is from the diploid to the tetraploid state, through a doubling of the chromosome set. This change is followed by a stepwise loss of chromosomes from the tetraploid cells resulting finally in a population of cells which are either hyper-triploid or hypo-tetraploid.

Summary

Cytological studies on experimental tumours growing *in vivo* or *in vitro* have revealed that the cell populations are heterogeneous in respect of chromosome constitution, and that the extent of deviation from the normal diploid state varies from tumour to tumour. It was observed that the stemline which represents the major numerical component of the cell population, is flexible; it may vary with time and is also influenced by environmental conditions.

Chapter 5

Chromosomal and Functional Differences
in Malignant Cell Populations

Biologists have put forward the view that the heterogeneous population structure of tumours enhances their progression. The chromosome variants in a tumour represent a pool of cell types with altered genotypes which confer certain advantages in a changing environment. Many studies have been carried out attempting to clarify the possible relationship between certain characteristics of tumours and chromosome patterns representing a particular genotype. Some of the findings from such studies are described below.

(1) *Drug resistance:* This is a very important practical problem in cancer therapy and any relevant information which may be obtained through the use of experimental tumours in animals is a valuable contribution towards our understanding of the mechanisms involved. Studies on drug resistance of micro-organisms indicate that random mutations and selection by particular drugs give rise to resistant variants from which stable populations of micro-organisms become established. Many experimental tumours have been tested against a variety of drugs, most of which are used in clinical practice, and resistant tumour sub-lines have been obtained. Their chromosome constitution was compared with that of the drug sensitive sub-lines and in some instances differences were observed. It was found that the modal chromosome number of an amethopterin resistant sub-line of Ehrlich ascites was 77 while that of the sensitive sub-line was 72; furthermore, the karyotype of the former contained two metacentric marker chromosomes which were absent from the cells of the sensitive sub-line (HAUSCHKA, 1958). In the L1210 murine leukaemia the very distinct submetacentric marker chromosome present in nearly every cell of the amethopterin sensitive sub-line was absent from the cells of the drug-resistant sub-line. On the other hand, resistance of these leukaemic sublines to azaserine, mitomycine and 5-fluorouracil was not associated with any particular chromosome pattern (BIESELE et al., 1961).

The chromosomal difference in amethopterin resistant sub-lines of Sarcoma-180 is shown in Fig. 14.

These sub-lines were developed by exposing the cell population of the parental tumour to increasing doses of the drug which seemed to select resistant cell variants present in the parental tumour. Since the number of these variants is small in the neoplastic population a very large number of cells had to be exposed to the drug for a considerably long time in order to develop a resistant sub-line (HAKALA and ISHIHARA, 1962).

In the murine lymphoma P388, 5-fluoro-deoxyuridine (5-FUDR) resistant sub-lines were obtained and subsequently maintained through *in vitro* culturing in a medium containing the drug, (YOSIDA et al., 1968). The chromosomal characteristics of the sensitive and resistant sub-lines are shown in Table 10.

The data suggests that the reduction in modal number is due partly to centric fusion of telocentric chromosomes and partly to the loss of whole chromosomes in

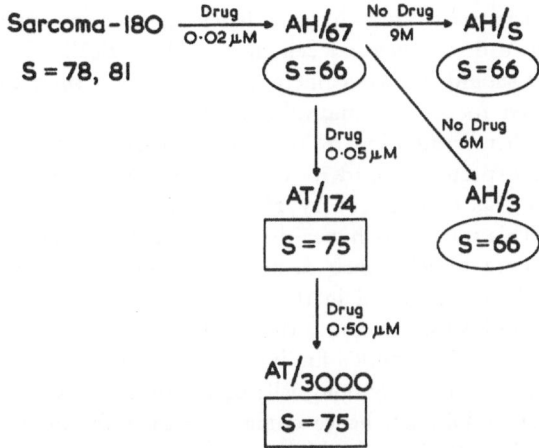

Fig. 14. Chromosome number of stem cells (S) and the degree of amethopterin resistance in Sarcoma-180 and its sub-lines. Sub-lines AH/S and AH/3 were derived from the 67-fold resistant line (AH/67) after having been grown in the absence of the drug for 9 and 6 months respectively (After HAKALA and ISHIHARA, 1962)

Table 10. Chromosomal characteristics of 5-FUDR sensitive and resistant sub-lines of lymphoma P388. (After YOSIDA, 1968)

Tumour sub-lines	Modal number	Percent of cells with modal number	Number of metacentric markers in modal cells
sensitive	49	26	14
resistant	40	52	21

the resistant sub-line. As in the experiment of HAKALA and ISHIHARA, resistance to 5-FUDR developed in a step-wise manner involving both mutation (represented by chromosomal change) and selection.

The above examples were chosen to illustrate the association of drug resistance with a particular chromosome constitution, and how the genome alteration involved in the development of drug resistance can consist in the loss or gain of chromosomes. There are many instances however, in which no chromosomal differences between sensitive and resistant sub-lines of tumours have been observed, e. g. the chromosomal patterns of both sensitive and resistant sub-lines of YOSHIDA ascites to a nitrogen mustard derivative were found to be identical; three clones of a murine fibroblast cell-line cultured *in vitro* and resistant to 8-azaguanine had the same chromosome number and pattern of variation as in the drug sensitive parental cell-line (YOSHIDA, 1968). These instances show that resistance to drugs can be conferred on cells with no detectable change in chromosome constitution. Similarly, it has also been reported that drug resistance of tumour sublines has been lost with no chromosomal change.

(2) *Radiation resistance:* Injuries to chromosomes by ionizing radiations are usually lethal to the cell. The damage consists of breaks in the chromosomes and the loss of acentric chromosome fragments during subsequent mitosis. In a diploid cell the loss of chromosome parts results in gene deficiencies which seriously impair cellular metabolism and leads to eventual cell death. Theoretically, it may be assumed that polyploid cells should be less vulnerable to radiation since chromosome losses could be compensated for by the multiplicity of homologous chromosomes. If this would be the case then irradiation of tumours containing both diploid and polyploid cells could be expected to lead to an increase in the proportion of the latter. Such an experiment was carried out by HAUSCHKA (1958) using the murine lymphoma of DBA/2. This tumour is hyper-diploid (modal number = 44) but contains three per cent of polyploid cells (their chromosome number varying between 84 and 90.) The lymphoma was irradiated in the animal (2,500 rads) without altering the proportion of polyploid cells, indicating that they were just as sensitive to radiation as the near-diploid cells. HAUSCHKA's finding can be explained by the work of other investigators who found that polyploid cells of tumours rarely contain exact duplicates of the original diploid set, hence damage to their chromosomes could not be compensated for by the extra homologues.

Some alterations in the chromosome pattern of BP8 sarcoma was achieved in my laboratory by exposing the ascites tumour to a total of 4,900 rads during 13 successive passages; the nature of the radiation induced changes is shown in Fig. 15.

Cytological analyses showed that while the modal chromosome number remained stable, the range of chromosome variation was reduced and the cells with high chromosome numbers were preferentially eliminated. On the other hand, radiation-induced alterations in the modal chromosome number have been observed in sub-lines of the L-strain. Fig. 16 shows that the modal number was reduced (RHYNAS and NEWCOMBE, 1961).

Further study revealed that the radioresistant sub-line contained a large metacentric marker chromosome; no such chromosome could be identified in the karyotype of the sensitive sub-line (WHITFIELD and RIXON, 1961). In a well planned experiment, RÉVÉSZ et al. (1963) investigated the response to radiation of 12 clones of the hyper-diploid Ehrlich ascites; in eleven the modal chromosome number was 46, in one it was 90, and in order to avoid any interference from the host's immune reaction the tumour cells were grown in diffusion chambers. They found no consistent relationship between chromosome number and radio-sensitivity.

These instances illustrate the very variable effects of radiation on the cell populations of experimental tumours in some no chromosomal alterations were found, while in others the range of chromosome variation was altered, the modal chromosome number shifted and distinctive marker chromosomes appeared.

(3) *Transplantability:* As a general rule tumours can be transplanted into the strain of origin, their take and growth depending on the genetic identity of tumour graft and host. The restriction of transplantability is due to antigens located on the

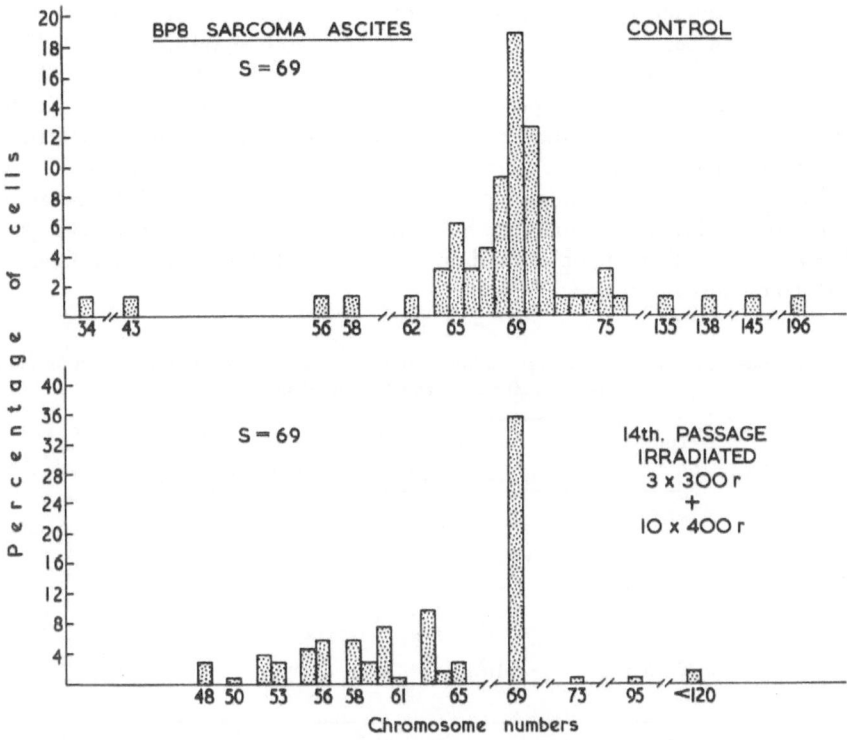

Fig. 15. Histogram showing the effect of radiation on the cell population of BP8 ascites
(By courtesy of Miss C. Talukdar)

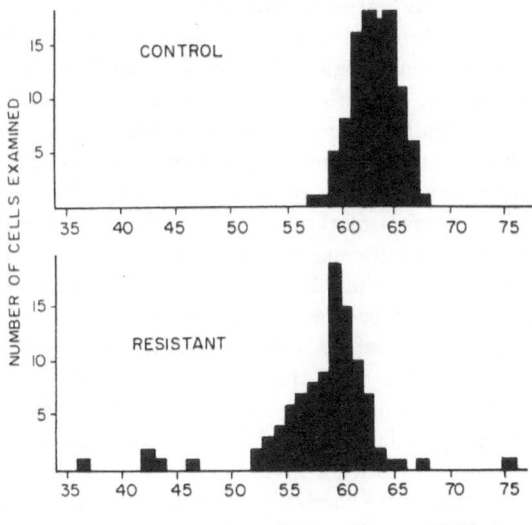

DISTRIBUTION OF CHROMOSOME NUMBER PER CELL

Fig. 16. Histogram showing the number of chromosomes in control and radioresistant sub-lines
of L-strain (Rhynas and Newcombe, 1961)

surface of the tumour cells and controlled by the *"histocompatibility genes"*. Fifteen such genes have been identified in the mouse, and most of them are located in the ninth linkage group. HAUSCHKA and LEVAN (1953) studied the behaviour of 25 mouse tumours in transplantation experiments and established a functional relationship between chromosome constitution and antigenic differentiation. They found that tumours with diploid or near diploid chromosome numbers are strain specific, while sub-lines of these tumours containing a high chromosome number could be transplanted into other (foreign) strains in which they were capable of progressive growth. Table 11 gives a few examples to show the relationship between transplantability and chromosome constitution.

Table 11. Modal chromosome number and immunogenetic specificity of murine ascites tumours (After HAUSCHKA and LEVAN, 1958)

Tumour	Strain of origin	Modal number	Transplantability into foreign strain
A/Lymphoma	A	44	none
		80	yes
6C3HED	C3H	40	none
		~46	yes
		~80	yes
Thymoma	DBA/2	42	none
		~85	yes

It is the general experience of research workers that during a long period of cultivation tumours become less antigenic, and this phenomenon is attributed to the fact that "antigenic cell variants" arise in the cell population by mutation (with or without alteration in the chromosome constitution), and these cells are able to "bypass" the foreign host's immunological defence system. Experiments in which antigenic cell variants could be identified were carried out by the KLEINS (1961) who found that while antigenically different variants isolated from two murine sarcomas had individually characteristic chromosome patterns, yet paradoxically in another case they were found to have the same chromosome constitution.

The immunological reaction of the host affects the growth rate and transplantability of a tumour. The chromosomal aspect of this process has been studied in the hypo-diploid Yoshida ascites, which has two large metacentric marker chromosomes (YOSIDA, 1968). During serial passage a third marker chromosome appeared which was submetacentric, and therefore easily identifiable. YOSIDA found that the transplantability and growth rate of the tumour increased in parallel with the rise in the number of cells exhibiting this new karyotype. The comparative proliferative capacity of various cell populations can be tested by mixed inoculation of the tumours into the same animal; such an investigation was carried out with two clones of Ehrlich ascites. In clone-1 the modal number was 47 and included a metacentric marker while in clone-2 it was 45 and included two markers. When the cells of the two clones were mixed together, or mixed with cells of the parental tumour and then injected into mice, cells from clone-2 proved superior to both the parental tumour and clone-1 as regards growth potential; this may be attributed to a greater proliferative capacity of the new karyotype, or to a lower antigenicity whereby cells of clone-2 could escape the host's immunological surveyance.

Results obtained in transplantation experiments have led to the conclusion that the ability of tumours to transgress strain barriers seems to be correlated with the departure of chromosomal constitution from the diploid state, and that there is a direct relationship between the degree of heteroploidy and transplantability. Examples described above show however that there are exceptions from this generalization, e. g. the murine carcinoma: TA3. This tumour originated spontaneously and had 40 chromosomes identical in every respect with the diploid karyotype of normal cells,

Table 12. Chromosome constitution and enzyme activities in HeLa variants
(After Bottomley et al., 1969)

HeLa-Sub-lines	Modal cells		Enzyme activity[a]			
	Chromosome number or range	Frequency	AP	LDH	G-6PDH	6-PGDH
A	74—84	—	0.003	1.7	0.44	0.08
229	79—81	—	0.10	0.9	0.30	0.08
S3G	75	38.0	0.740	0.3	0.68	0.11
	79	50.0	0.740	0.3	0.68	0.11
G	69	62.0	0.120	2.6	0.15	0.05
	71	34.0	0.120	2.6	0.15	0.05
65	65	68.0	0.006	1.6	0.12	0.05
71	71	66.0	0.560	2.5	0.10	0.06
75	75	64.0	0.410	1.9	0.55	0.07

[a] Enzyme activity estimation: AP: μmoles of p-nitrophenol formed min/mg protein; LDH: μmoles of NAD converted to NADH min/mg protein; G-6PDH: μmoles of NAD converted to NADPH min/mg protein; 6-PGDH: μmoles NADP converted to NADPH to min/mg protein.

and could only be transplanted into strain A mice, which was the strain of origin. A sub-line of this tumour designated as TA3Ki is hypo-tetraploid with a modal chromosome number of 69 including two metacentric markers, and this sub-line retained its transplantation specificity. However another sub-line (TA3Ha) gained one extra autosomal chromosome (modal number = 41) and was not only successfully transplanted into six foreign strains of mice, but also proved lethal to rats from four strains. This particular tumour, though near-diploid and only slightly deviant from the diploid karyotype had lost its strain specificity in transplantation (Hauschka et al., 1971).

(4) *Metabolic variation:* Bottomley and co-workers (1969) used seven metabolically different sub-lines of HeLa to investigate the relationship between biochemical differences and chromosome constitution. The biochemical characteristics of the sub-lines were shown by the enzyme levels of alkaline phosphatase, glucose-6-phosphate dehydrogenase, lactic dehydrogenase and 6-phosphogluconic dehydrogenase and their modal chromosome numbers are given in Table 12.

Alkaline phosphatase levels show the greatest variation from cell-line to cell-line, the largest being a 200-fold difference between HeLa/A and HeLa/S3G; variations in the other enzyme levels lie within much narrower limits. These differences may stem from point gene mutations, or from gross chromosomal alterations which can then be observed, although there is not always a consistent relationship between these structural and functional changes. Similarly, no correlation could be established between chromosome constitution and metabolically variant sub-lines of the secondary clones of L-strain (HSU and KELLOG, 1959). On the other hand some correlation has been detected in four plasma-cell leukaemias of mice (FJELDE et al., 1962) and three clones of Chang liver cell-lines showed variations in alkaline phosphatase activity which seemed to be correlated with differences in chromosome constitution (see Table 13).

Table 13. Chromosome constitution and alkaline-phosphate activity of CHANG liver clones
(After KÖNIGSBERG and NITOWSKY, 1962)

Modal number of chromosomes		Clone 4	Clone 6A	Clone 8A
		65	70 (M)[a]	75 (M)
Alkaline phosphatase	Specific activity[b]	0.1	10.5	45.8
	Thermal stability[c]	Stable	Stable	Inactivated

[a] Marker chromosomes present
[b] μmoles p'nitrophenol liberated in 30 minutes at 38°C
[c] at 56°C

"Minimal deviation hepatomas" represent examples of the earliest stages of malignant transformation which are available in transplantable form (VAN POTTER, 1964). Thirty-five such hepatomas in various stages of "deviation" from the normal were analysed by NOWELL et al. (1967). It was expected that the larger the biochemical deviation from normal, the greater the change in chromosome constitution of the liver cells. However, cytological studies failed to demonstrate such a correlation, as all 29 hepatomas with aneuploid chromosome numbers had different karyotypes with no obvious relationship between specific chromosomal aberrations and enzyme changes; amongst six diploid hepatomas two were found to be more biochemically deviant from normal than tumours with aneuploid chromosome constitutions.

Progression of hormone dependent tumours to autonomy may be accomplished with or without chromosome changes; thus HELLSTRÖM (1961) found autonomous sub-lines of a hormone dependent testicular tumour in mice had chromosome patterns similar to their dependent parental tumour. Yet distinct chromosome differences between hormone dependent adenocarcinoma of the rat thyroid gland and its hormone independent sub-line were reported by AL-SADI and BEIERWALTERS (1967) who found the modal chromosome number to be 42 in the former (including one marker chromosome present in only two per cent of cells), while the hormone independent carcinoma had a modal number of 40 (including the marker chromosome present in 70 per cent of cells). The growth rate of the autonomous tumour was fourteen times higher than that of the hormone dependent carcinoma.

Summary

The studies described above illustrate how experimental tumours, their sub-lines and clones may differ in various characteristics e. g. resistance to drugs, antigenicity, enzyme activities and hormone dependence and that in some there is a correlation between biochemical parameters and chromosome constitution while in others there is not. This paradoxical situation reflects the complexity of the relationship which exists between the number and morphology of the chromosomes and the functional expression of the genome, which cannot always be directly correlated with the visible chromosome constitution. However, the most important value of these experiments is in providing further proof that the cell populations of tumours contain variants of various kinds, adapted to certain functions, and under particular circumstances they can be selected to replace the original cell composition of the tumour. The origin of cell variants is through mutation; the mutant cells may be identified by chromosomal changes, but very often they lack phenotypic characteristics and their presence can only be detected by selection experiments.

Chapter 6

Primary Tumours in Animals

The principles which are assumed to govern the behaviour of malignant cell populations have been derived both from cytological studies of experimental tumours passaged *in vivo,* and from cell-lines grown *in vitro.* The tumours used in these studies were transplanted for many generations so their cell populations became far removed from the original, and therefore could not be considered to be representative of tumours generally. In the following part, the chromosome constitution and behaviour of *primary* tumours will be considered and the findings compared with those obtained from investigations on experimental tumours.

Studies aiming to determine the chromosome constitution of primary tumours are beset with many difficulties, partly due to technical reasons and partly to the fact that at the time of the cytological analysis the chromosome variants observed may represent only one phase in the evolution of the malignant cell population. Another difficulty arises from the presence of non-malignant stromal cells which cannot be distinguished from tumour cells if the latter have a diploid chromosome set containing no structurally altered chromosomes. Furthermore, it should be realised that cytological analyses fail to reveal *"microstructural"* changes in the chromosomes, and yield no information concerning the process of malignant transformation of cells at the gene level.

The forthcoming part deals with the chromosome studies of tumours arising "spontaneously" or induced by various agents. The former represent malignancies, the causal agents of which are not at present known.

1. "Spontaneous" Primary Tumours

BAYREUTHER (1960 a) studied twelve mammary adenocarcinomas in mice, nine of which were diploid and three hyper-diploid. Similar observations were made by OHNO et al. (1959) who analysed seven mammary carcinomas developed in Swiss mice; in one tumour every cell was diploid, in another the modal number was 41, and the remaining five tumours had both diploid and hyper-diploid cells. The cytology of "spontaneous" leukaemias in mice has been studied by STICH et al. (1959) and BAYREUTHER (1960 a); while the latter found only diploid cells in 28 out of 32 murine leukaemias, the former workers observed hyper-diploidy with modal numbers of 41 and 44.

2. Induced Primary Tumours

(1) *Endocrine imbalance:* Hormone dependent pituitary tumours in seven male mice were found to have the normal diploid chromosome number. During a course of serial implantation into pre-conditioned animals, two tumours became hormone independent; one retained the diploid stem line, while the other developed a new stem line of 65 chromosomes including three long metacentric markers. Out of nine mammary tumours induced by hormonal imbalance, and supposedly virus-free, eight were diploid and one hyper-diploid (BAYREUTHER, 1960 b).

(2) *X-radiation:* Ford and his associates (1958) carried out extensive cytological studies on 60 leukaemias and related malignancies in mice, all induced by ionizing radiations. They analysed the leukaemic cells at the primary and metastatic sites as well as in transplants. The chromosome numbers in one radiation induced leukaemia (modal number = 41) is shown in Table 14.

Table 14. Chromosome numbers in spontaneous and X-ray induced leukaemias in mice
(After FORD et al., 1958)

Leukaemia	Sites	Chromosome number							Total no of cells
		$\leqq$39	40	41	42	43	44	45+	
Spontaneous in	Marrow	7	4	—	4	4	29	1	49
AK-strain	Spleen	1	1	—	21	3	12	1	39
	Thymus	1	—	—	1	1	13	1	17
	M*node	—	—	—	4	2	8	2	16
	A*node	—	1	1	29	1	5	1	38
Total		9	6	1	59	11	67	6	159
X-ray induced in	Marrow	6	38	6	—	—	—	—	50
C57Bl-strain	Spleen	3	30	67	—	—	—	—	100
	M*node	1	—	23	1	—	—	—	25
	Pt*nodes	1	—	13	10	1	—	—	25
Total		11	68	109	11	1	—	—	200

M*: mesenteric; A*: axillary; Pt*: paratracheal

For comparison Table 14 also includes the findings obtained from a spontaneous leukaemia in AK-strain, in which the distribution of chromosome numbers is bi-modal, one peak being at 42 and the other at 44. Those cells with 44 chromosomes predominate in the bone marrow and thymus, while those with 42 are mainly located in the axillary lymph node. Both cell types have a small acrocentric marker chromosome. In the radiation induced generalized leukaemia the modal chromosome number was 41. The cells with 40 chromosomes could be normal stromal cells, however the presence of a very small acrocentric chromosome in a few cells with 40 chromosomes suggested that at least some of these cells were leukaemic. Cytological analyses also revealed different chromosome constitutions in the various tissues, e. g. in the marrow 76 per cent of cells had 40 chromosomes, while in the spleen the predominant cell type (67 per cent) contained 41 chromosomes. Similar analyses were made on leukaemic cells in the primary and secondary hosts into which the leukaemia was transplanted. The findings of one such study is given in Table 15.

The distribution of chromosome numbers was bi-modal in the spleen; this pattern was maintained in the 5th. and 7th. transplants in the spleen but not in the axillary lymph node where the frequency of cells with 41 chromosomes became reduced to 4.2 while those with 43 increased to 78.7 per cent. The difference in the frequency of cells with 41 and 43 chromosomes between the lymph node and the spleen is of statistical significance ($\chi^2 = 10.46$). According to FORD and co-workers the high frequency of the 43 chromosome type in the axillary lymph node can either be attributed to "an adaptive preference for that anatomical environment or to the chance of early seeding of the site by a 43 chromosome leukaemic cell". The first alterna-

Table 15. Chromosome constitution in primary leukaemia and its transplants. (After FORD et al., 1958)

Tumour	Site	Chromosome no.		Total no. cells
		41	43	
Primary	spleen	21.8[a]	36.3	55
5th Transplant	spleen	25.2	33.6	107
7th Transplant	spleen	27.6	53.1	47
	axill. node	4.2	78.7[b]	47

[a] per cent

[b] stem line cells with 43 chromosomes are favoured in the node, the difference between spleen and axillary node is very significant ($\chi^2 = 10.46$)

tive is considered to be the most likely one. FORD and his associates found that nine of the 60 leukaemias were mostly composed of cells with 40 chromosomes, and these were indistinguishable from the chromosomes of normal diploid cells. The range of deviation from the diploid number was found to be narrow, the number of extra chromosomes in leukaemic cells varying between one and five. New chromosome types due to structural alterations were observed in 23 leukaemias, but no clone of cells with the same altered chromosome was found. Out of the 60 cases of leukaemia analysed one had a modal number of 80.

(3) *Chemical carcinogens:* Fourteen subcutaneous sarcomas induced by methylcholanthrene administration in mice were studied by HELLSTRÖM (1959); ten tumours were diploid and the other four were hyper-diploid. Other investigators found hyperdiploid and hyper-tetraploid modal chromosome numbers in methylcholanthrene induced tumours, and made the interesting observation that tumours of the latter type had a long latent period, while those with near diploid chromosome constitutions had a short one.

By intraperitoneal administration of Freund's adjuvant, fourteen plasma cell tumours were induced in mice. Three were diploid with a few cells containing 80 chromosomes; one was hyper-diploid and the cells of the other ten had near tetraploid chromosome sets (MORIWAKI et al., 1969). One of the diploid tumours was transplanted into new hosts where the diploid chromosome constitution changed to near tetraploid in the second transplant generation. Fig. 17 illustrates the transformation of the diploid tumour.

The cytology of 30 tumours induced by chemical carcinogens in mice, rats and hamsters was studied by BAYREUTHER (1960 a), who found the modal chromosome number to be diploid in 20 tumours.

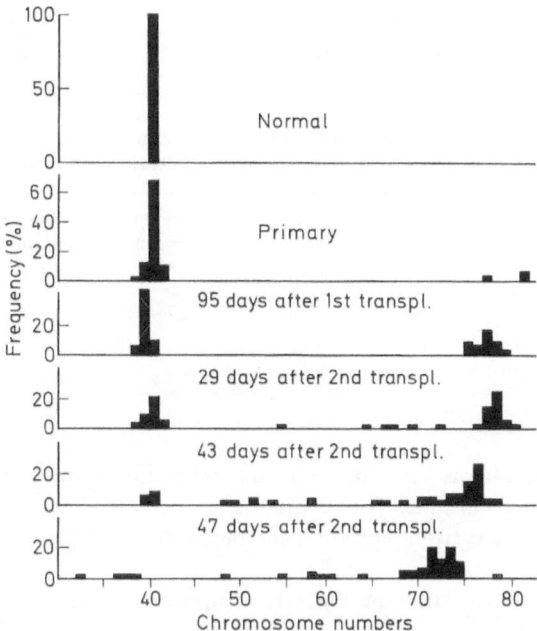

Fig. 17. Alteration of chromosome number in a mouse plasma cell tumour during transplantation; in the second transplant the near-diploid cells were replaced by cells with hypotetraploid chromosome number (MORIWAKI et al., 1969)

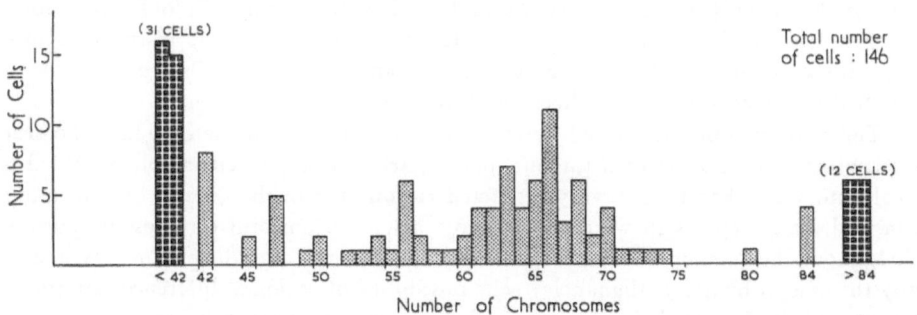

Fig. 18. Histogram showing the chromosome numbers and their frequency in a rat sarcoma induced by imferon (By courtesy of Dr. A. J. S. DAVIES)

Imferon, an iron dextran drug used in clinical practice until it was discovered to be carcinogenic, produces sarcomas in rats mainly at the site of injection. The chromosome constitution in one such tumour is shown in Fig. 18.

The frequency of diploid cells with 42 chromosomes was only five per cent, the majority of cells containing more than this number. While the range of chromosome variation was wide, the frequency of each chromosome variant was low, some being represented by only a single cell; therefore, even though the modal chromosome number was 66, only eleven cells of the 146 cells analysed contained this number. Tumours induced by the administration of p-dimethylamino-azobenzene in the liver of rats were studied by YOSIDA and ISHIHARA (1958). The proportion of diploid cells observed in four independent hepatic nodules of the same liver, and the range of chromosome variation is shown in Table 16.

Table 16. The frequency of cells with diploid chromosome number and the range of chromosome variants in four hepatic nodules in a rat. (After YOSIDA and ISHIHARA, 1958)

Liver lobes	Nodules	Percentage of 2N-cells[a]	Range of variation in chromosome number
II	A	29.0	25—151
II	B	75.0	27— 78
III	C	40.0	34—168
III	D	96.0	—

[a] 100 cells were analysed in each nodule

Tumour nodule D was diploid, while the other three contained a mixed population of chromosome variants. This finding is a very important one, since it demonstrates that in the same tissue environment neoplastic cell populations can develop independently.

Another kind of variation in the cell composition within the same tumour is illustrated by Fig. 19.

The chromosome number was determined in cell samples taken from six different regions of a primary sarcoma induced by imferon in the rat. The histogram shows the chromosomal differences found between the six samples. Out of a total of 150 cells analysed, only three cells from sample V had the normal diploid chromosome number. Cells with 83 chromosomes constituted the "largest" group in the six samples, with a frequency of 13.5 per cent; karyotyping of these cells from sample V revealed that several contained dicentric chromosomes.

The two examples described above show the difficulty in determining the true chromosome constitution of a tumour, particularly when the cell sample analysed is small and was taken from a very restricted region. Yet in the general literature one can find many reports in which the authors assume a uniform chromosome pattern throughout the tumour, some of which may be of very large dimensions (as is usually the case in human malignancies); the possibility of regional differences are thereby completely disregarded. Changes in chromosome constitution have also been observed in cell samples taken at different times from the same tumour; in view of such findings a chromosome pattern may represent only a particular situation which exists in a certain region of the tumour at a specific time. Before a "stable" pattern is established, cellular instability can persist for a long period of time, during which mitotic disorders introduce more numerical and structural changes in the chromosome pattern of the malignant cell population.

An extreme case of such cellular instability was investigated by the author in a primary sarcoma induced by aromatic mustard in the rat (KOLLER, 1953). The tumour contained a very high number of mitotic abnormalities of various kinds, the most conspicuous anomaly being chromosome bridges, shown in Fig. 20 a and 20 b.

The abnormal chromosome behaviour was analysed in the primary tumour and followed in the cell populations of 93 transplants. The frequency of cells with chro-

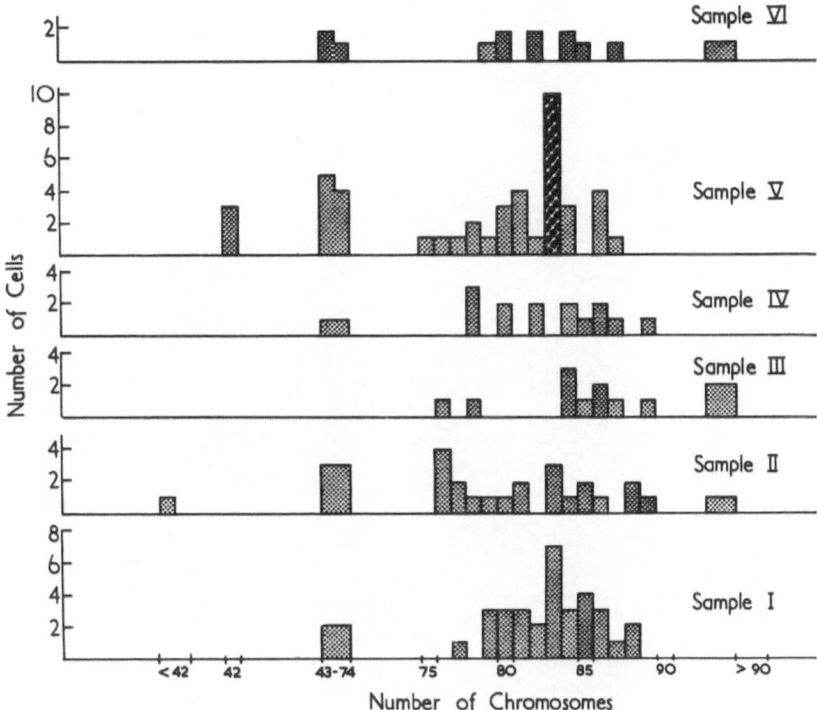

Fig. 19. The different chromosome numbers and their frequency in cell samples taken from six different regions of a rat sarcoma, induced by imferon (By courtesy of Dr. A. J. S. DAVIES)

mosome bridges was 68.5 per cent in the primary tumour, in the last transplant it was reduced to 16 per cent. The number of "bridges" in single cells, their length and configuration exhibited a wide range of variation. Fig. 21 illustrates the types of anaphase bridges observed in the primary tumour.

Some cells were found to be free of chromosome bridges, some had only one while in others their number increased to ten or even more. The diagram of Fig. 22 shows the various stages of chromosome changes leading to the formation of anaphase bridges.

The initial event is breakage in the chromosome filament, which occurs during interphase, this is followed by rejoining the ends of the broken chromosomes into a new configuration. At anaphase of the successive mitosis the centromeric part forms the dicentric single strand bridge which may break at telophase, and the broken chromosome forms a new dicentric in the interphase nucleus, as shown in the diagram. Depending on the locus of break in the chromosome bridge, the "break-fusion-bridge" cycle can yield bridges of different lengths. New chromosome types e. g. rings, quadriradials and minutes were also seen in the tumour cells. The modal chromosome number was 56 and the frequency of cells containing this number was 12

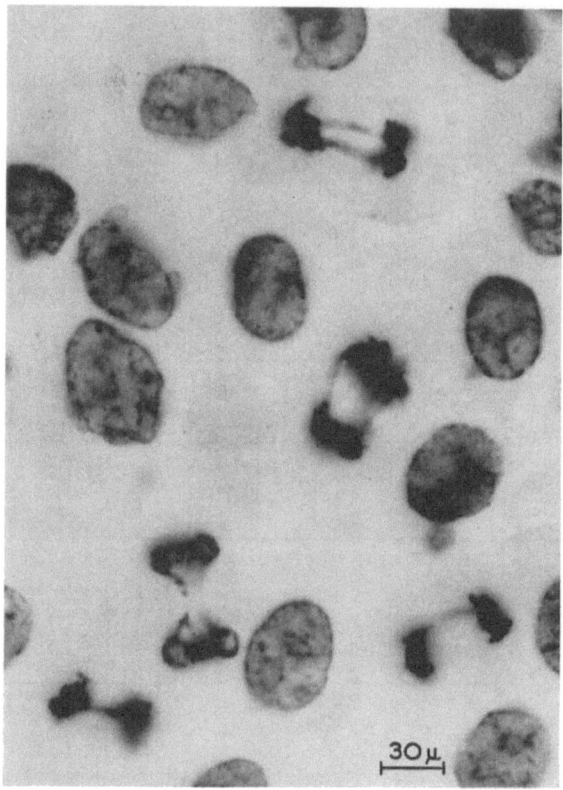

Fig. 20a

Fig. 20. Chromosome bridges in a rat sarcoma induced by nitrogen mustard; a) five dividing cells with chromosome bridges; b) nine microphotographs of ana- and telophases showing various types of chromosome anomalies

per cent. Cells with more than 84 chromosomes (4N) were also observed but they were rare.

The relationship between the frequency of abnormal mitoses and the growth rate of the tumours was studied at various stages of transplantation. It was found that the greater the growth rate of the tumour (as measured by its size increase within a definite period), the lower the proportion of cells with mitotic anomalies, and *vice versa;* such an inverse relationship was to be expected, but it was not always the case. Sister tumours derived from the same parent tumour but developed in different rats, very often showed significant differences in growth rate and fre-

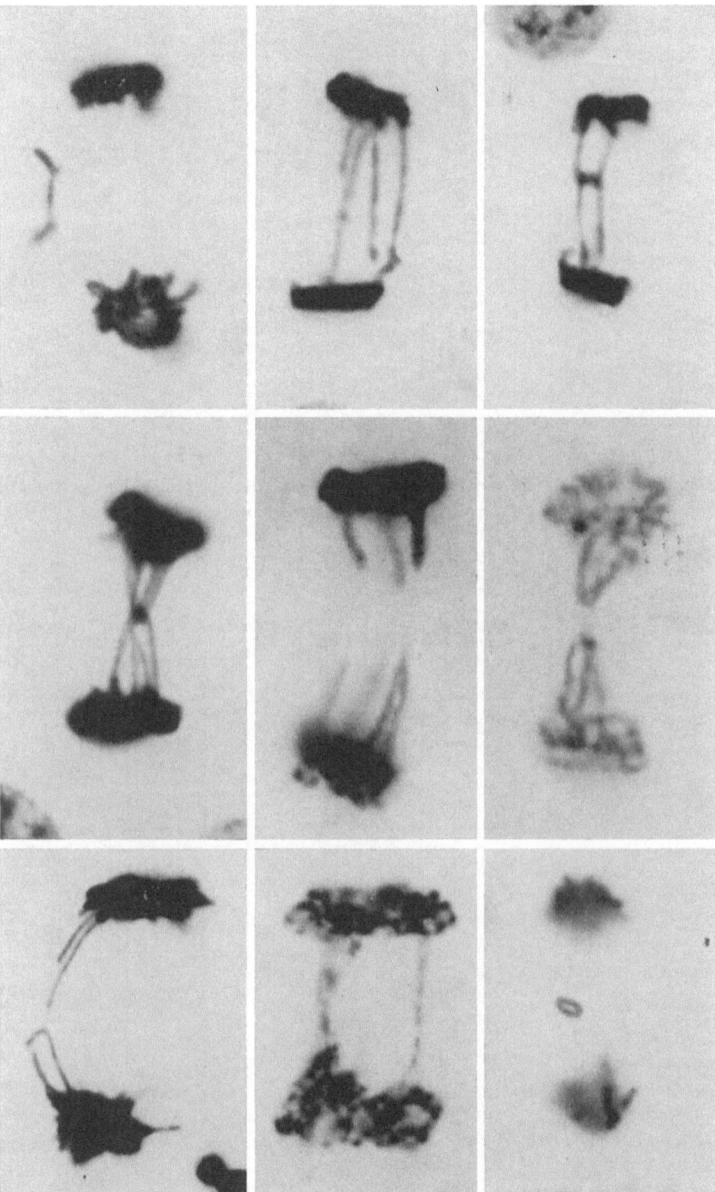

Fig. 20b

quency of mitotic aberrations. This may either be attributed to differences in the cell composition of the grafts or to differences in the immune response exerted against the tumour by the host animals, which were only "colony-bred" and hence not genetically identical. Differences in growth rate however were also observed in sister tumours which had developed in the same animal, and it is therefore very likely

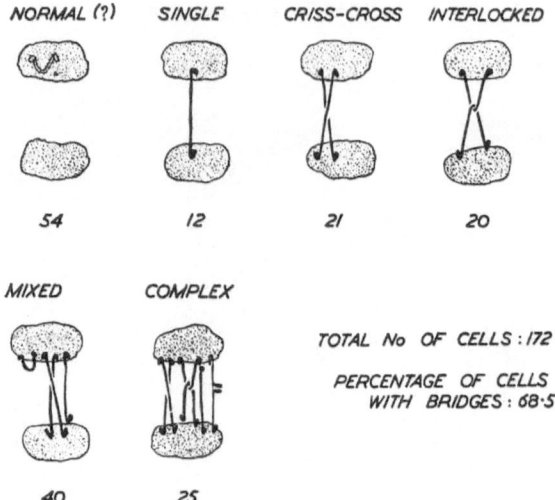

Fig. 21. Diagram showing the distribution and types of anaphase bridges in the primary sarcoma induced by nitrogen mustard

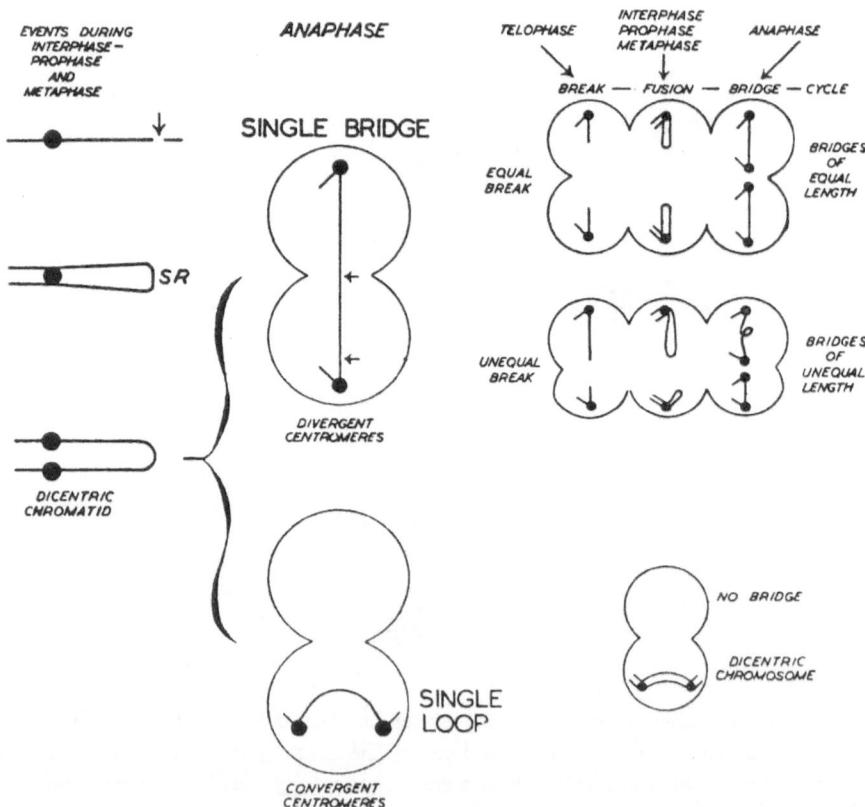

Fig. 22. Diagram illustrating the origin of anaphase chromosome bridges

Table 17. Cytological characteristics of nitrogen mustard induced tumours in the rat

Compound	Tumour	No. of Transplantation	Cytological features			Duration	% of mitotic abnormalities
			Anaphase Bridges	Fragments	Polyploidy		
CB 1048	A	93 Gen	+++	+	+	Permanent	16.8
	B	10	+	+	+	Temporary	5.6
	C	7	—	—	++	Temporary	8.0
$N(CH_2CH_2Cl)_2$	D	0	—	+	—		not analysed
	E	2	++	+	+	Temporary	6.0
	F	8	—	—	—	Normal	nil
	G	3	+	+	+	Semi-Permanent	12.6
CB 1047	A	0	—	+	+		3.2
	B	0	—	—	++		9.5
$N(CH_2CH_2Cl)_2$	C	0	—	—	—		nil
	D	7	+	—	+	Temporary	3.0
	E	4	+	++	+	Temporary	4.5
	F	0	—	+	+		7.5
CB 1044	A	0	++	—	—	"Localised" chromosome stickiness	18.0
CH_3 — $N(CH_2CH_2Cl)_2$	B	0	—	+	+		2.0
	C	2	+	+	—	Temporary	not analysed
	D	0	—	—	—		nil
	E	2	—	—	+		7.0

that the cause lies in the different degrees of cellular instability of the transplanted cell population. This has been demonstrated in an experiment where tumour cells of the 35th. transplant generation were cultured *in vitro*, and dividing cells in the culture were followed by cinephotography. In the culture no cells with anaphase chromosome bridges were found, yet when these cultured cells were re-transplanted into animals and a tumour developed, cells with chromosome bridges re-appeared (KOLLER and WAYMOUTH, 1952). It seems that the expression of cellular instability is under the influence of the environment, *in vivo* it persisted up to the 93rd. transplant generation. The cytological study of this particular tumour shows that structural and numerical alterations in chromosome constitution can arise in malignant cells not only in the initial phase of tumour development, but at any stage in the growth of the tumour. It seems that cellular instability can persist for a long period of time in tumours, and results in the variable spectrum of chromosome patterns and behaviour.

The type, frequency and constancy of chromosomal anomalies in 18 primary tumours induced in rats at the site of injection by three related nitrogen mustards have been determined, and the data are shown in Table 17.

Only three tumours were found to be free of mitotic aberrations; several of the primary tumours containing cells with mitotic aberrations were transplanted into new hosts, and most of the tumours which subsequently developed were free of the aberrations seen in the parental tumour.

(4) *Virus-induced primary tumours:* Nineteen mammary carcinomas of a strain of mice known to harbour the mammary tumour virus were analysed by TJIO and ÖSTERGREN (1958); the chromosome constitution was diploid (40) in 16 tumours, and the frequency of such diploid cells was nearly 100 per cent. One carcinoma was hypo-diploid with a stem line of 39 chromosomes; another had two stem lines, one was diploid and the other tetraploid; their frequencies were 58 and 42 per cent respectively; the last tumour was tetraploid, 92 per cent of the cells karyotyped had 80 chromosomes, and the other 8 per cent contained 79—81 chromosomes. On transplantation of the carcinomas the chromosome constitution remained the same in the new hosts.

The chromosome constitution of virus-induced tumours was analysed in four species of animal (fowl, mice, rat and rabbit) by BAYREUTHER (1960 a). He found that erythroleukaemia in the domestic fowl consisted of cells with the characteristic diploid chromosome number of the species (12 macro-chromosomes and about 60 micro-chromosomes). Similarly, in sarcomas induced by the Rous agent in mice, cells with the diploid chromosome number formed the dominant class (MARK, 1967 and KATO, 1968). The analysis of 76 tumours induced by GRAFFI, GROSS, FRIENDS, MTA (mammary tumour agent) and Shope virus showed that in 75 the modal number was the diploid chromosome number. It seems that the chromosome pattern in virus-induced tumours is nearly identical with that of normal cells. These malignancies form a distinct category of their own and in view of recent discoveries in this field of cancer research, the relationship between chromosome constitution and oncogenic viruses will be discussed in more detail in Chapter 12.

Summary

The examples described above illustrate the general pattern of chromosome behaviour in primary tumours of animals; the tumours are basically of two kinds: one is composed mostly of cells with the diploid chromosome constitution, the other is characterized by a cell population which contains a great number of chromosome variants deviating from the diploid condition. This deviation may be small e. g. X-ray induced leukaemias, or large e. g. chemically induced sarcomas, and very often no mode can be identified. The chromosome pattern of early primary tumours, particularly those with a diploid modal number, very frequently undergo progressive alteration in chromosome constitution during the later stages of tumour development. The incidence and extent of chromosomal changes increase with time. Cytological studies have shown that primary tumours are individual in respect of (1) chromosome number, (2) spectrum of chromosome variants (3) frequency of cells with different chromosome numbers and (4) marker chromosomes. Tumours induced by the same carcinogenic agent may vary in their cytology. Cellular instability, as indicated by mitotic aberrations can persist for long periods (particularly in chemically induced tumours). The chromosome pattern of primary malignancies can become stabilized, and as such can be carried over into transplants without change, though instances are also known when this is not the case. The chromosomal characteristics of primary malignancies in animals show a great degree of similarity to those observed in experimental tumours which have been maintained by transplantation for long periods of time.

Chapter 7

Chromosome Aneuploidy in Human Malignancies: Effusions

Cytological studies of experimental ascitic tumours in mice and rats have shown that free cells in the peritoneal fluid provide very suitable material for chromosome analyses, and their behaviour can be manipulated in experiments. Furthermore, it was observed that the ascitic fluid represents an environment in which malignant cells are independent, and can express unhindered their potentialities as regards proliferation and chromosome variability. The cytological findings in ascites tumours of animals stimulated similar studies into the effusions of cancer patients.

The early reports described single cases; thus Hsu (1954) analysed the chromosomes of a metastatic melanoma obtained from the peritoneal effusion of a patient and cultured *in vitro*. Hsu counted the chromosomes in a sample of 92 cells and found a range of variation from 40 to 100, the greatest proportion of cells having less than 65 chromosomes. HANSEN-MELANDER et al. (1956) analysed cells of the peritoneal ascites of a patient whose carcinoma of the ovary was being treated with radiotherapy, and observed variations in the number of chromosomes in their cell sample similar to those found by Hsu, and reported that the modal number was 58. Using improved cytological techniques these and other early studies clearly demonstrated that malignant cell populations in man contain chromosome variants, thus confirming the findings of HANSEMANN, BOVERI and WINGE.

The conditions existing in human malignant effusions differ greatly from those found in the ascites of mice and rats. In the former the tumour cells are not derived from an inoculum of free cells, but either from a distant primary site or from metastatic adhesions growing on the serous membranes of the peritoneum or pleura. The malignant cells in effusions exhibit several characteristics of morphology and behaviour which are not commonly observed in tumour tissue. The present author investigated the chromosomes in 98 effusions obtained from 58 patients with carcinoma of the ovary, breast, bronchus and bladder, and some suffering from Hodgkin's disease. My report described the chromosomal variability in the cell population of peritoneal and pleural effusions, and discussed the cause and evolutionary significance of chromosome polymorphism in the development of tumours (KOLLER, 1956). Cell samples were collected from ascitic fluids by centrifugation; the amount of fluid aspirated at each paracentesis varied from 0.5 to 12 liters. It was found that patients differed in the rate of retention of ascitic fluid, in some it was very high and within a few days several liters of fluid accumulated. The density of cell populations in the large volume of fluid was extremely low and no reliable estimates of the number of cells present could be made. Whilst significant differences were found in the viscosity of the various ascitic fluids, only slight variations were observed in pH. Most of the effusions contained not only malignant cells but also benign cells e. g. macrophages, polymorphonuclear leukocytes and mesothelial cells present in varying proportions. Usually degenerating cells were also encountered in the ascitic fluid, their number depending on the "age" of the effusion. The cell composition of the ascitic fluids was found to undergo continuous alteration in the proportion of the various cell types and the number of degenerating cells. The cellular changes are believed to be due to alterations in the physiological and nutritional condition of the effusions.

Differences in the cell composition were observed between the peritoneal and pleural ascitic fluids. Thus it was found that pleural effusions contain many types of inflammatory and mesothelial cells of the serous membranes, making up about 30 per cent of the total cells in the fluid; on the other hand the cell composition of the peritoneal effusions was more uniform, benign cell types being rare and constituting less than 5 per cent of the cell population.

The malignant cell population of human ascitic fluid consists of isolated cells and aggregates (see Fig. 23 a and b).

The aggregates are of two types; one is composed of cells with indistinct boundaries, the other contains cells with definite cell membranes. The number of nuclei in a cell colony may be as high as 200, but the average number is around 80. The diameter of the nuclei varies from 7 μ to 35 μ reflecting differences in their chromosome content. It was found that the malignant cell population in the pleural fluid was usually of the "free-cell" type while in the peritoneal cavity the "cell-colony" type was the most common.

The chromosomes were counted in 212 cells sampled in six cancerous effusions, their number varied between 25 and 150; the most common numbers were between 50 and 65. The incidence of mitotic anomalies was found to be high, and consisted of multipolar spindles, over-contraction of metaphase chromosomes, anaphase chromosome bridges and superfragmentation or complete disintegration of chromosomes (see Fig. 24 a, b, c, d, e, and f).

Binucleate cells are of common occurence in effusions, the nuclei present may differ in size and their division is not always synchronized. Dividing binucleate cells were observed in which the chromosomes of one nucleus were in the process of disintegration. Giant cells in division, with hundreds of chromosomes have also been encountered, occuring more often in "old" effusions. The quantity and quality of the ascitic fluid and the time interval between successive paracenteses were found to be the factors which affect the mitotic apparatus.

The chromosome constitution in effusions of the same patient was compared in cell samples taken at different occasions. In five of nine such cases studied, the chromosome pattern, range of variation and the number of cells with the same chromosome number were similar; in the other four instances the cell population of the successive effusions showed significant differences in chromosome patterns.

Since fluid from the body cavities can not be completely removed by aspiration, a variable amount of the "old" fluid with its cell population remains, hence chromosome constitutions similar to those observed in the cells of the previous effusion can be expected, provided the environmental conditions remain the same. The appearance of new chromosome patterns observed in successive effusions may be the result of selection of chromosome variants present in the previous effusion and favoured

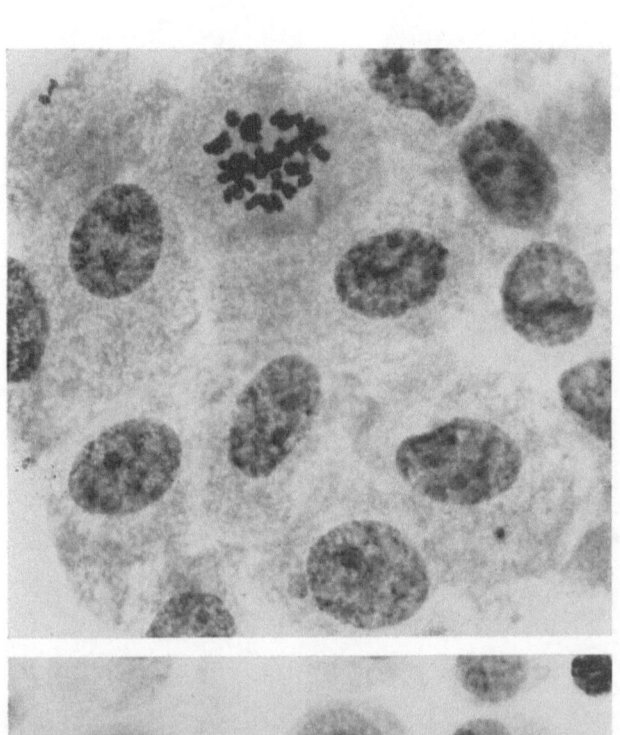

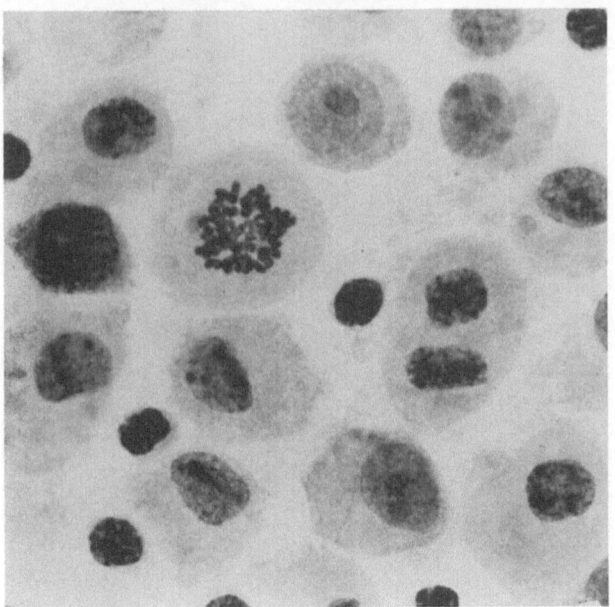

Fig. 23. Malignant cells in human ascitic fluid: a) "free-cell" ascites with one binucleate cell and two cells with a micro-nucleus; b) section of a "cell-colony" in which cell boundaries are indistinct

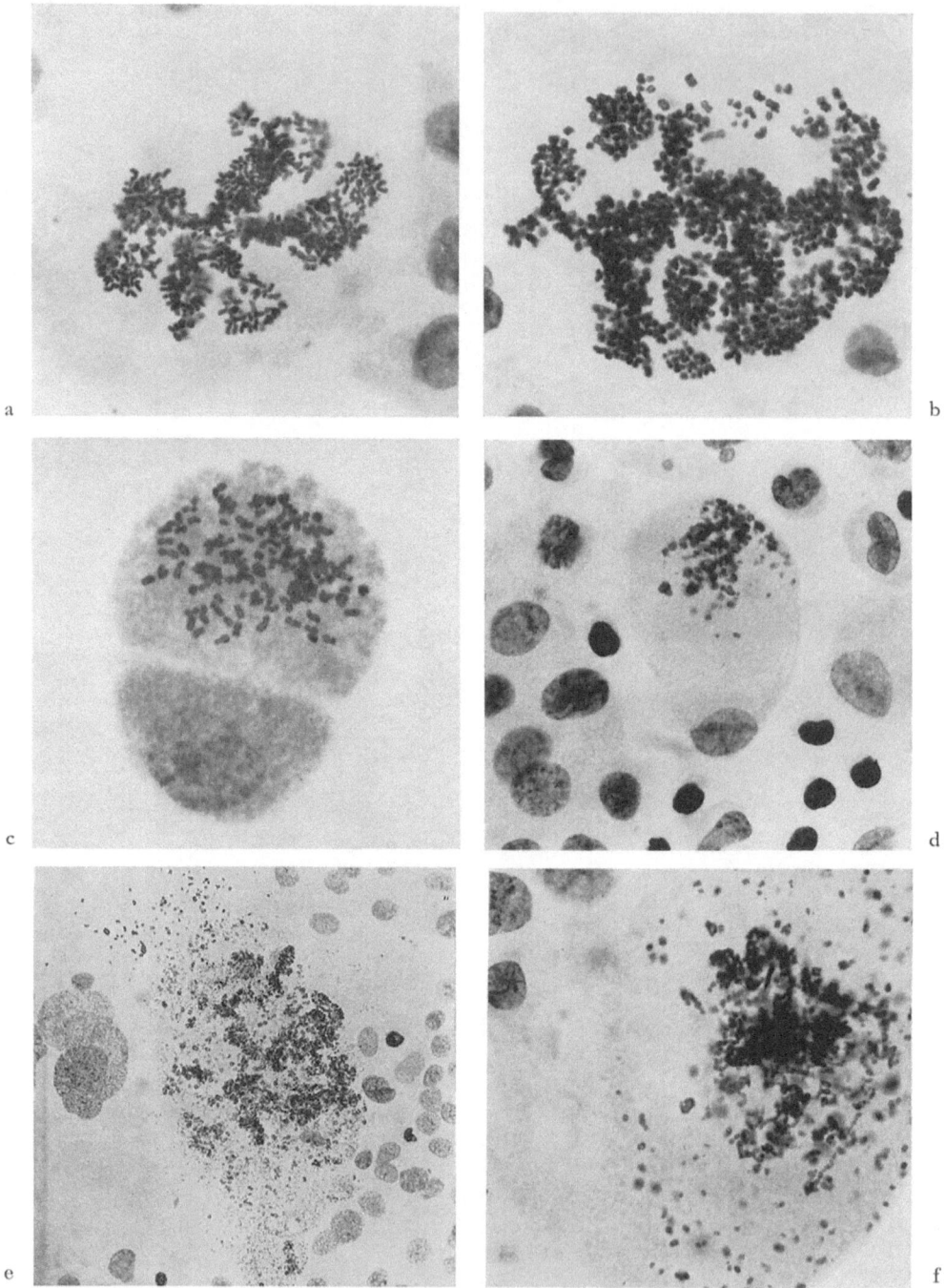

Fig. 24. Mitotic anomalies: a) multipolar metaphases; b) multipolar spindles in dividing giant polyploid and multinucleate cells; c) mitosis in a "doublet"; d) abnormal binucleate cell in which only one nucleus has entered mitosis; e) chromosome disintegration in a giant cell; f) superfragmentation of the chromosomes, the acentric fragments are scattered in the cytoplasm, while the centric chromosome segments form several groups on the equatorial plate

by the physiological conditions of the new environment. However, the different chromosomal patterns of the new cell population may be due to the introduction of cells shed from the metastatic adhesions on the serous membranes and containing chromosome constitutions not represented in the preceding effusion. Such an event may have occured in one of our patients who had a peritoneal effusion; although the time interval between the two paracenteses was only four days, the cells sampled had very different chromosome patterns.

During my studies on human carcinomatosis, twelve patients were seen with double ascites; one in the peritoneal and the other in the pleural cavity. The chromosome constitution of malignant cells in the effusions at the two sites were very similar, with one exception; in this particular patient the post mortem investigation revealed the presence of two carcinomata; one was adenocarcinoma of the uterus and the other lymphosarcoma of the nasopharynx, and it was assumed that the significant differences in chromosome constitution between the cell populations of the two effusions were the result of having been derived from the two different primary tumours. It is not improbable however, that the gross chromosomal differences observed between the peritoneal and pleural effusions in the above case, were due to environmental differences existing at the two sites.

Table 18. Modal chromosome number and range of variation in five human ascites
(After MAKINO et al., 1959)

Primary Tumour	Metastatic Site of Ascites	Total number of cells	Modal number	Percentage of modal cells	Range
Reticulosarcoma	Pleural	32	46	31.2	41—49
Breast carcinoma	Pleural	100	75	48.4	69—79
Gastric carcinoma no. 1	Peritoneal	111	74	43.0	73—77
Gastric carcinoma no. 2	Peritoneal	42	72	21.4	68—79
			76	14.3	
Gastric carcinoma no. 3	Peritoneal	201	42	21.3	40—49
			45	14.4	
			84	10.0	76—87

The present author's investigations also provided evidence that the "fluid" environment can not be considered to be the cause of malignant cell behaviour. A benign peritoneal effusion was found in one patient with a pathological liver lesion; the ascites was of the "free-cell" type and contained a high number of degenerating cells, as well as several dividing cells all with the diploid chromosome number. While in malignant ascites chromosomally abnormal cells survive and proliferate, in benign ascites such cells degenerate and die. Several similar observations were made by other investigators. Since the ascitic fluid is the ideal medium in which malignant cells can express their capacity for change and adaptation, it provides a suitable material in which to observe the mechanisms responsible for chromosome variation. Through studies of effusions the present author reached the conclusion that in this medium the progression of cancer cells towards full malignancy is both enhanced and accelerated.

Further evidence that chromosomal heterogeneity is a characteristic feature of malignant cell populations was provided by MAKINO and his associates (1959) who analysed the chromosomes of 30 human ascites tumours. Five cases were selected from the 30 studied, since the cell samples analysed were large enough to yield meaningful information. The modal chromosome number and range of variation of these effusions is shown in Table 18.

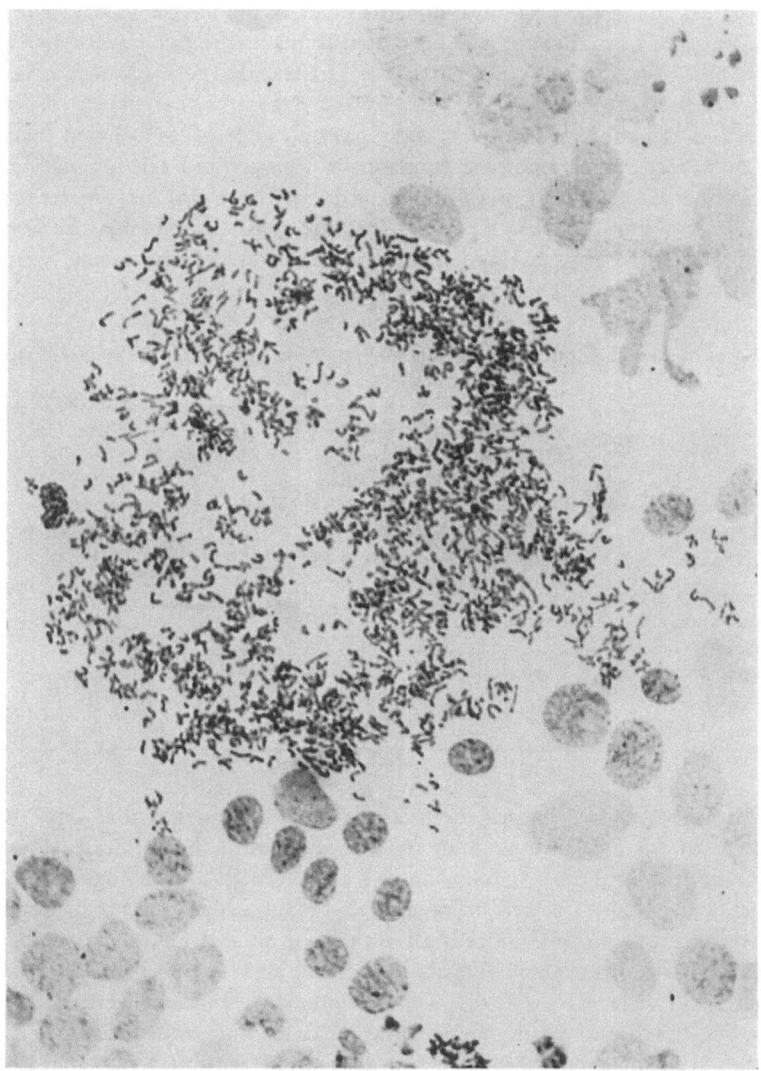

Fig. 25a

Fig. 25. a) Dividing cell with approximately 800 chromosomes; b) karyotype of a malignant cell from a pleural effusion; the number of chromosomes is 130 and include 6 marker chromosomes

These cases illustrate the general pattern of variation encountered in their studies, and show that the karyotype of tumours deviates from the normal. Each tumour has its own karyotype differing from that of other tumours including those which originated in the same organ. Further data from another survey in which 52 human ascitic tumours were investigated led the authors to the conclusion that variation in the number and morphology of chromosomes is a characteristic phenomenon of human cancer (MAKINO et al., 1964).

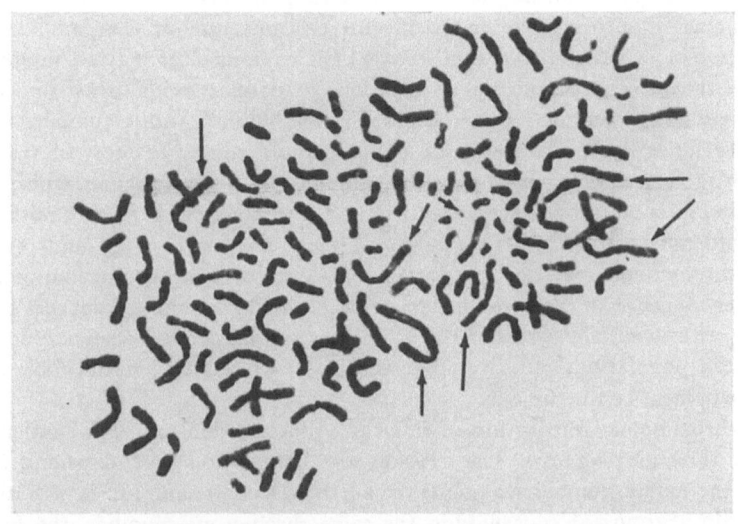

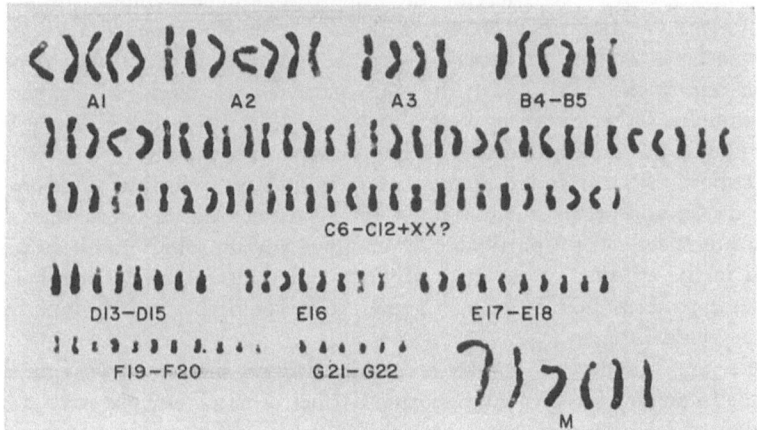

Fig. 25 b

More detailed and extensive chromosome studies of malignant effusions were carried out by Dr. A. A. SANDBERG and his associates at the Roswell Park Memorial Institute, Buffalo. The reports published by these investigators deal with various aspects of chromosomal behaviour in cell populations of human ascites. They contain data concerning the extent of chromosome variability in particular groups of tumours; chromosomal variation within a single tumour sampled at different occasions; a comparison of cell behaviour in malignant effusions and benign ascites; identification of chromosomes in abnormal karyotypes and a special study of malignant cells with a normal diploid chromosome number (ISHIHARA et al., 1961; ISHIHARA, 1962; ISHIHARA and SANDBERG, 1963; SANDBERG, 1966; SANDBERG et al., 1963, 1967, 1968 a, b; SANDBERG and HOSSFELD, 1970). Their main finding was that in contrast to the sharp modes of 46 in non-malignant effusions there was a considerable spread in the chromosome number of malignant effusions, all of which were characterized by an abnormal modal number ranging from 39 to 133, with no particular number more prevalent or specific for any one tumour. The modal cells constituted not more than 30 per cent of the cells examined. It was an interesting observation that a high proportion of effusions in patients with breast or ovary carcinoma had modal numbers in the diploid range, while in other tumours the modal number was usually in the hypo- or hyper-triploid range. In most of the effusions analysed by SANDBERG's group new chromosome types were present which were not represented in the normal karyotype; the origin of the "marker" chromosomes however, could not be traced with certainty. Though the morphology and incidence of marker chromosomes varied from case to case, an acrocentric chromosome two to four times longer than chromosomes of group D in the human karyotype, was found in many effusions. The presence of ring chromosomes and dicentrics observed in various cell populations indicates that chromosomal rearrangements took place during development of the tumour.

The chromosome constitution of one cancerous effusion has been studied in more detail by these investigators. The effusion was sampled on four occasions, and variation in the modal number was observed in the different samples. It was also found that within a group of cells having the same chromosome number, the karyotypes were different. The frequency of cells with marker chromosomes also varied; in the cell sample taken at the last occasion, two large marker chromosomes were present in 90 per cent of the cells, though the same markers were much less frequent in earlier cell samples. Other instances were also reported, in which no significant variation in chromosome patterns was observed in successive cell samples of the same ascitic fluid. SANDBERG's team found that the karyotypes of cancerous effusions are relatively stable, and when shifts occured in the chromosome pattern they could be attributed to selection of a particular chromosome variant which had been previously observed in the effusion. When two effusions had the same modal number and the chromosome patterns in this group of cells were compared, it was found that the karyotypes were different.

In the large number of human ascites studied no similar karyotypes could be identified. In a few effusions the majority (80 per cent) of malignant cells had normal diploid chromosome constitutions; the range of chromosome variation around the mode was narrow and no cells with high polyploid numbers were present. However, in other cases with diploid modal numbers, karyotyping revealed several of the cells with 46 chromosomes to be "pseudo-diploid" i. e. the karyotype contained morphologically abnormal chromosomes. Effusions were encountered in which more than 50 per cent of the cells contained over 600 chromosomes, and in one cell more than 1000 chromosomes were counted. Similar observations of cells with extremely high chromosome numbers were made by the present author, and are illustrated in Fig. 25 a and 25 b.

SANDBERG and his colleagues found that in ascites containing cells with high chromosome numbers, the modal number was well below 92: the tetraploid number of human chromosomes. When cells from this particular effusion were cultured *in vitro*, the chromosome number in dividing cells was in the hypo-tetraploid range and no cells with polyploid chromosome constitutions were seen in mitosis. It seems that in the altered environment the latter could not divide.

SANDBERG and his co-workers made a survey of the cytological findings published up to 1966, and summarized the frequency distribution of modal chromosome numbers in 129 cancerous effusions.

Table 19. Distribution of modal chromosome number in 129 cancerous effusions
(SANDBERG et al., 1967)

Chromosome Constitution	Modal Range	Percentage of Cases
Diploid Range		
Hypo-	35—45	17.0
Pseudo-	46	14.0
Hyper-	47—57	17.0
Total		48.0
Triploid Range		
Hypo-	58—68	15.5
Pseudo-	69	0.8
Hyper-	70—80	23.3
Total		39.6
Tetraploid Range		
Hypo-	81—91	6.2
Pseudo-	92	0.0
Hyper-	93—133	6.2
Total		12.4

Table 19 shows that in the cases studied, the largest number of effusions have a modal number within the diploid range (35—57). When however, the individual groups were separately analysed, effusions with a hyper-triploid modal range were found to be the most common. The extensive studies of the SANDBERG-group have established the fact that chromosome aneuploidy is a characteristic feature of cell populations in cancerous effusions of man.

The sources of cells in the ascitic fluid are the "solid" growths of tumours located at distant sites in the body. The environment of the two cell populations differ greatly and it might be argued that chromosome behaviour of the "free" cells living and multiplying in a "fluid" medium, cannot be representative of the cells which exist in the primary tumours. The next chapter describes findings from analyses of chromosomes in *solid* tumours, and attempts to clarify further the relationship between these tumours and the metastatic effusions, revealed by their chromosome patterns.

Summary

The fluid of human malignant effusions provides an extremely suitable medium in which cancer cells can fully express their basic potentialities. Cells of malignant effusions have the following general characteristics: (1) modal chromosome numbers widely deviant from the normal diploid state, (2) a small proportion (less than 30 per cent) of modal cells, (3) a wide range of chromosome variation, (4) no identifiable fixed, stable stem-line, (5) a high frequency of mitotic anomalies and finally (6) a cell population which changes with time. On the other hand, cell populations of benign ascites always have a well defined diploid mode and few chromosome variants.

Therefore, in spite of gross chromosomal aberration the very viability of malignant human effusions reveals the proliferative advantages of such a chromosomally heterogeneous cell population.

Chapter 8

Chromosome Aneuploidy in Human Malignancies: Solid Tumours

Chromosome studies of malignant cell populations in "solid" tumours of man are more difficult than those of the free cells in effusions, due to technical difficulties and the scarcity of dividing cells in biopsy material. Before 1956 a few observations had been made concerning abnormal chromosome constitution and behaviour in tumours, but no comparative cytological analysis of groups of human malignancies had been carried out. In a report considered to be "the earliest karyological characterization of human neoplasms" (Hsu, 1961) the present author described chromosome · behaviour in a hypo-diploid adeno-carcinoma. The chromosome number in this particular tumour showed a great variation, cells with 36, 32, 24 and 16 chromosomes being the most numerous. Synchronous division of groups of adjacent cells was frequent. Chromosomes and occasionally whole chromosome sets were found to fragment, as shown in Fig. 26.

The viability and proliferative capacity of these hypo-diploid cells led me to the conclusion that adjacent tumour cells are dependent on each other (KOLLER, 1947 a).

The first study to describe chromosomes in a series of solid tumours in man on a comparative basis was that of MAKINO and his associates (1959). Through the use of an improved cytological technique these investigators obtained metaphases with better fixed and stained chromosomes, and could thus count their number and identify the position of the centromere in each chromosome. The characterization and comparison of chromosome patterns in different tumours was made possible by following the method of TJIO and LEVAN (1956) who had arranged the human chromosomes of cancer cells into the following three morphological groups: (1) M-group having median or sub-median centromeres (2) S-group with sub-terminal centromere and (3) T-group having a terminal or near terminal centromere.

The report of MAKINO et al. (1959) contained the cytological findings of nineteen solid tumours at seven different sites. The data presented in Table 20 is a sample of their findings.

The difficulty encountered in the cytological study of biopsy material is indicated by the small number of cells in which the chromosomes could be analysed. Some tumours contained more than one modal number, and using the karyotyping method of TJIO and LEVAN (1956) MAKINO et al. analysed the cells of three such tumours, (one mammary and two uterine). Their results are given in Table 21 which shows numerical changes occuring in all three chromosome types.

The authors found no correlation between the abnormal chromosome constitution and the histo-pathological structure of the tumours.

Their comparative study indicates a general pattern characterizing the chromosome constitution of human malignances. Tumours in which the chromosomes could be counted and analysed in a large number of cells exhibited the following trends: (1)

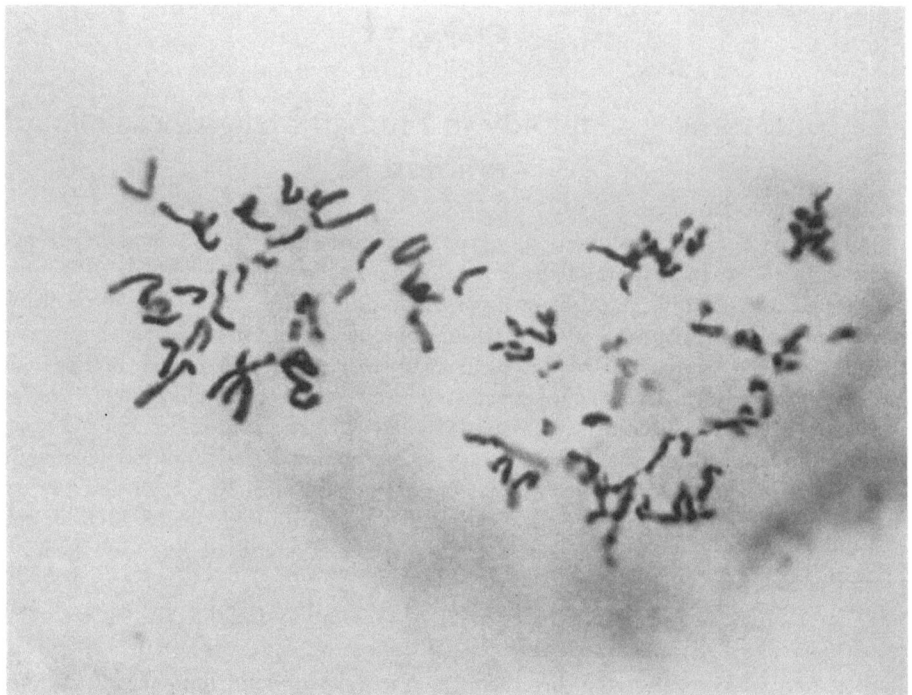

Fig. 26. Two hypo-diploid metaphases, one showing fragmentation of chromosomes

a wide range of variation in chromosome number in each tumour (48—120); (2) the range of variation in chromosome number differed between tumours; (3) the number of chromosomes deviated from the normal diploid number; (4) tumours originating in the same organ had different chromosome constitutions; (5) morphologically altered chromosomes (i. e. differing in size and shape from those in the normal karyotype) were observed in many tumour cells, including those in the modal group. The authors drew the conclusion that "the chromosome number of human primary tumours varies within a wide range, being wider than in transplanted tumours of rats and mice".

HAUSCHKA surveyed the karyological findings published up to 1960 concerning more than a hundred human tumours (mainly malignancies of the haematopoietic system), and found that the presence of abnormal chromosome constitutions far exceeded the chromosome patterns indistinguishable from the normal diploid human karyotype; in an excellent address at the Symposium of the American Association for Cancer Research in 1960, he discussed the possible significance of chromosome

Table 20. Chromosome variability in solid tumours. (After MAKINO et al., 1959)

Tumours	Major range of variation	Modal number	No. cells analysed
Maxillary ca. (M1)	64— 78	71 (33.3)[a]	13
Maxillary ca. (M2)	69— 78	73 (38.4)	13
Maxillary ca. (M3)	63—104	none	13
Maxillary ca. (M4)	66— 80	69 (38.4)	13
Gastric ca. (Gs1)	55— 58	56 (40.0)	5
Gastric ca. (Gs7)	89—112	none	5
Gastric ca. (Gs8)	108	none	3
Skin ca. (no. 26)	48— 54	53 (56.2)	16
Urethral ca. (no. 30)	83— 87 (45—120)[b]	84 (30.0)	23

[a] Numbers in brackets indicate the percentage of cells with the modal chromosome number
[b] Number indicates chromosome variants beyond the major range of variation

Table 21. Multiple modes and chromosome constitution in two tumour types
(After MAKINO et al., 1959)

Tumours	Total no. of cells	Major range	Modes	Chromosome types		
				M	S	T
Normal karyotype	—	—	—	20	20	6
Mammary ca. (M2)	47	56—72	58 (8.8)[a]	29	23	6
			65 (19.1)	32	27	6
			69 (12.8)	32	30	7
Uterine ca. (Ut5)	56	44—54	50 (17.8)	22	24	4
			51 (54.0)	22	24	4[b]
Uterine ca. (Ut3)	42	43—58	48 (19.0)	22	20	6
			55 (14.0)	20	25	10

[a] Percentage of cells with modal number
[b] Minute extra chromosome is present

aneuploidy in normal development and cancerous growth (HAUSCHKA, 1961). Evidence of numerical and structural alterations in the chromosome constitution of cancer cells was provided by SPRIGGS and co-workers (1962), who studied primary tumours of the cervix, brain and lung; They found a wide range of aneuploidy and abnormal chromosomes e. g. rings, dicentrics within the same tumour. The presence of similar structurally abnormal chromosomes in more than one cell led them to the conclusion that these cells are derived from a single progenitor and represent a clone.

The morphological characterization of human karyotypes made it possible to compare individual chromosomes of cancer cells with those in normal cells, and to identify the extra chromosomes in aneuploid metaphases. Following this procedure, MAKINO et al. (1964) karyotyped modal cells in several uterine and mammary carcinomas; a sample of their results is shown in Table 22.

It can be seen that every chromosome group is affected, the increase in chromosome number being greatest in the C-group. These investigators found many of the addi-

Table 22. Karyotypes in modal cells. (After MAKINO et al., 1964)

Tissue	Modal number	Chromosome-Groups							marker chromosomes
		A	B	C+X	D	E	F	G+Y	
Normal	46	6	4	14+X	6	6	4	4+Y	—
Tumour									
Uterine ca. (U61)	44	6	4	16	6	5	4	3	—
Uterine ca. (U63)	52	7	5	23	3	6	6	1	—
Uterine ca. (U73)[a]	77	8	7	⌐———— 56 ————⌐				4	2 min[b]
	86	8	7	⌐———— 65 ————⌐				4	2 min
Mammary (Mm78)	60	7	4	27	5	6	4	4	3 sub[c]
Mammary (Mm79)	72	11	5	30	6	9	4	5	1 sub and 1 min

[a] bimodal
[b] 'minute' chromosome
[c] long subterminal chromosome

Table 23. Range of chromosomal variation. (From ATKIN and BAKER, 1966)

Tumours	Range of chromosome numbers	No. of cells analysed
Cervix ca. No. 7	41—43	3
Cervix ca. No. 8	41—44	9
Cervix ca. No. 5	44—48	53
Cervix ca. No. 12	47—48	3
Cervix ca. No. 15	51—52	4
Cervix ca. No. 3	55—61	59
Uterine ca. No. 10	46[a]	50
Uterine ca. No. 11	46—47	13
Uterine ca. No. 13	48—50	6
Uterine ca. No. 16	53—54	5

[a] several cells were "pseudo-diploid"

tional chromosomes could be matched with chromosomes of the normal karyotype, and that structurally altered "marker" chromosomes could also be identified. By using the "marker" chromosome present in modal cells, ATKIN and BAKER (1966) were able to indicate the possible sequence of events occuring during the development of new cell types; in the cases studied these events involved loss of identifiable chromosomes. The study of these investigators also revealed that the range of chromosomal variation in tumours within the same organ was narrow, and grouped around the modal chromosome number (see Table 23).

A more detailed cytological study was carried out by YAMADA et al. (1966) who analysed the chromosome constitution in seventeen solid tumours, and found great diversity in the karyotypic pattern of the various tumours, no tumour being diploid and no two tumours having similar karyotypes. In the majority of tumours they identified altered marker chromosomes, the number and morphology of which varied from tumour to tumour. It was also noted that none of the tumours analysed had

Table 24. Range of modal chromosome number in 91 human primary tumours and in 129 malignant effusions. (SANDBERG and HOSSFELD, 1970)

	Range	Percentage of Cases primary	effusions
Diploid:			
Hypo-	35—45	17	17
Pseudo-	46	9	14
Hyper-	47—57	35	17
Group Total		61	48
Triploid:			
Hypo-	58—68	12	16
Pseudo-	69	2	1
Hyper-	70—80	14	23
Group Total		28	40
Tetraploid:			
Hypo-	81—91	10	6
Pseudo-	92	1	0
Hyper-	93—133	0	6
Group Total		11	12

tetraploid modal chromosome numbers, the percentage of cells with modal chromosome numbers represented only a minor proportion of the total cell population.

These early reports illustrate the progress in the analyses of chromosome constitutions in solid tumours of man. The studies first established the fact that aneuploidy i. e. deviation from diploidy, is a characteristic feature of cancer cells, which reveal great variability in modal number. Karyotypic analysis, when it could be applied, demonstrated that the frequency of changes occuring in particular groups of human chromosomes is variable, and drew attention to the clonal evolution of chromosome aneuploidy. The chromosome constitution and behaviour in solid tumours have been found to be very similar to those observed in the malignant cell populations of effusions. SANDBERG and HOSSFELD (1970) collected data from reports published before 1967, and their findings are given in Table 24, which shows the range of variation in the modal chromosome number in the two kinds of malignancies: primary tumours and effusions. They do not differ significantly from each other, except for the higher incidence of cells with very high ploidy in malignant effusions.

According to these authors the most striking feature of their survey is the absence of "diploid" tumours. While the diploid chromosome constitution in solid tumours and effusions is rare (MILES, 1967) it is of common occurence in leukaemias, other malignant haematopoeitic disorders and tumours either caused by or associated with viruses. These groups of malignancies will be considered in future chapters.

Summary

Aneuploid chromosome constitution in solid tumours is a general phenomenon. Deviation from the normal pattern of chromosome composition is variable, the range stretching from hypo-diploidy to hyper-tetraploidy. It has been found that cells of the stemline represent only a small proportion of the total cell population; instances were observed in which no modal chromosome number could be identified, while in others two modes were present. Analysis of cells with 46 chromosomes showed many of these cells had "pseudo-diploid" karyotypes. Cells with the same number of chromosomes frequently contain different karyotypes. Comparison of chromosome constitution in a large number of solid tumours has shown that in the majority the modal number is hyper-diploid, and the range of chromosome variation lies between 47 and 57. Marker chromosomes are present in most tumours, though their morphology and frequency vary greatly in the cell populations. Morphologically similar marker chromosomes were observed in several cells within tumours, indicating a clonal origin of these cells from a common progenitor. Numerical changes affect all chromosome groups in the human karyotype, the greatest increases were found in group C. Karyotypes of primary tumours do not show a consistent pattern for any particular malignant growth. The great variability observed in the chromosome composition of neoplastic cells within the same tumour and between different tumours, together with the presence of diploidy in some tumours, seem to reflect the secondary nature of visible chromosomal changes in the malignant behaviour of cells.

Chapter 9

Marker Chromosomes and the Clonal Evolution of Chromosome Aberrations

Marker chromosomes are important since diploid cells with morphologically altered chromosomes can indicate the malignant nature of the cells, and the presence of similar marker chromosomes in different tumours may be used as one of the criteria by which particular groups of malignancies can be characterized.

The most studied marker chromosome is Ph' (Philadelphia chromosome) already referred to in previous chapters. This marker chromosome was discovered by No-well and Hungerford (1960) in blood cells of patients with chronic myeloid leu-kaemia (CML); it is one of the G-group chromosomes, and according to recent studies Ph' is identified as chromosome 22 (O'Riordan et al., 1971). Ph' chromosome differs from its normal partner by the loss of a great part of the long arm, and contains only 61 per cent of the DNA present in normal chromosome 22 (Rudkin et al., 1964). The deficient chromosome is restricted to the haematopoietic system, its presence has been demonstrated in the precursors of granulocytes, erythrocytes and megakaryocytes. Ph' is acquired during adult life, it is not constitutional or inherited, as shown by the case of monozygotic twins in which only the member of the pair with CML had the Ph' chromosome, (Goh and Swisher, 1965). The presence of Ph' in patients developing CML after radiation treatment also indicates that it is an acquired chromosomal defect. The chromosome has been found in over 90 per cent of reported cases of typical CML in both adults and children, but in rare instances it has also been seen in other diseases related to leukaemia. Thus Popp and Lizzi (1970) reported a case of acute lymphocytic leukaemia in which a high percentage of marrow cells contained the Ph'. In a few instances Ph' has been observed in the preleukaemic state without the characteristic clinical syndromes, it was present in the bone marrow cells but not in the granulocytes circulating in the blood (Kemp et al., 1963). In cases simulating CML e. g. myelo-fibrosis, the absence of Ph' is decisive in diagnosing the condition and in deciding on the treatment.

Cases of CML in which the Ph' chromosome is absent are of special interest. Studies of Ph'-negative cases of CML have shown that they form a heterogeneous group with poor prognosis and lack of response to treatment. The age of onset of Ph'-positive and negative CML shows significant differences. In a recent study of 223 CML patients the average age was found to be 45 years in Ph'-positive cases, and 60—65 years in Ph'-negative cases (Whang-Peng and Canellos, 1971). It is not improbable that the granulocytes of Ph'-negative CML have an abnormal G chromosome. Such a case has been reported by Schneider et al. (1967) who found the marrow cells to contain a metacentric G chromosome of apparently normal size in every metaphase karyotyped. The authors suggested that the abnormal chromosome originated by a pericentric inversion and is associated with a small deletion having clinical and haematological consequences identical to those of the Ph' chromosome.

The terminal stage of CML is usually associated or preceded by a "blastic phase" in which the chromosome pattern of leukaemic cells with Ph' undergo further changes. The chromosomal changes are not necessarily identical in different patients but have a tendency to form a uniform pattern. The appearance of two or more Ph' chromosomes usually coincides with the onset of the blastic phase (PEDERSEN, 1968). Hyper-diploidy is the most common type of aneuploidy which appears in marrow cells during blastic crisis. Cases are however also known, in which blastic transformation was not accompanied by further karyotypic changes (HAMMUDA et al., 1964).

The significance of the Ph' marker chromosome in CML has been extensively discussed by clinicians and research workers. The suggestion that the consistency and specificity of Ph' in CML indicates a *causal* relationship has been put forward by NOWELL and HUNGERFORD (1964); they argued that CML might result from a mutagenic agent acting within a single precursor cell in the marrow to cause a deletion and produce the Ph' chromosome, and that this chromosomal change confers a selective advantage on the cells which then overgrow the haematopoietic system. Perhaps information from future studies will provide a more tangible proof of the causal relationship between Ph' and CML, at present however, the true importance of Ph' lies in the fact that this is the first instance in which a specific chromosomal change is characteristic of a specific type of malignant disease in man. The Ph' chromosome is an important marker, it has prognostic value and serves as a useful criterion in evaluating response to treatment.

Cytological studies have been carried out on a large number of myelo-proliferative disorders, some believed to be variants of CML since they very often terminate in a similar clinical picture. One aim of these studies was to find out if consistent chromosomal abnormalities may be characteristic of other malignant conditions. SANDBERG and co-workers (1968 a) analysed the chromosome constitution in 219 cases of *acute leukaemia*, and found a very variable pattern; nearly 50 per cent of the cases had aneuploid modal chromosome numbers ranging from hypo-diploidy to hyper-tetraploidy, while the others apparently had diploid modes. These investigators also found that in cases of acute leukaemias with the same modal chromosome number, the karyotypes were different. Comparative karyotypic analyses of many cases seem to indicate that in acute leukaemia certain autosomes of group C are more frequently affected than other chromosomes.

In *erythroblastic leukaemia* ("Di Guglielmo" syndrome) no consistent or characteristic chromosomal changes were reported, aneuploidy mostly consisted of hypo-, pseudo- and hyper-diploidy, the latter was however quite rare (KIOSSOGLOU et al., 1965). Abnormal marker chromosomes have been observed by KROLL and SCHLESINGER (1970). The Ph' chromosome was encountered in a variant of erythroblastic leukaemia, which seems to suggest a relationship between this disease and CML (CASTOLDI et al., 1968)

Cytological studies of *polycythaemia vera* showed that chromosome constitution is apparently normal in the majority of cases, but progression into the leukaemic phase of the disease is usually associated with changes in the normal pattern, and in some cases with the appearance of Ph'. Many of the cells with 46 chromosomes were found to be pseudo-diploid, and the presence of an extra chromosome in the C group was observed in several cases (KAY et al., 1966). Apart from the random loss of C or F group chromosomes in some cases, no characteristic chromosome pattern or presence of a consistent marker chromosome could be established in *lymphoma, lymphosarcoma* and *reticulum cell sarcoma* (LAWLER et al., 1968). On the other hand, a consistent deletion in the short arm of a chromosome in group E has been reported in malignant lymphoma, follicular lymphoma and Hodgkin's disease by SPIERS and BAIKIE (1968 a) who suggested the term *"Melbourne chromosome"* to describe it. The presence of this marker chromosome was interpreted as evidence of a relationship between these three malignancies.

Table 25. Frequency of tumours with or without marker chromosomes. (After ATKIN, 1970)

Tumours		No. of Tumours with		No. of
type	numbers	identical "giant" marker	other markers	tumours without markers
Ca. Cervix	15	4	7	4
Ca. Uterus	7	7	3	17
Ca. Ovary	21[a]	13	7	1
Total	63	24	17	22

[a] including 15 peritoneal effusions

In several cases of *Waldenström's macroglobulinaemia* and *multiple myeloma* an extra abnormal chromosome, approximately the size of an A-group chromosome, was found. It should however be emphasized that the size and shape of this marker varies considerably not only in the different gammopathies, but in different patients with the same disease (HOUSTON et al., 1967). The possibility should also be borne in mind that morphologically similar marker chromosomes may differ in their genetic constitution. By using the quinacrine fluorescence staining method "internal" differences in morphologically similar chromosomes have been demonstrated (STEELE, 1971).

Cytological studies of malignant conditions in the haemato- and lymphopoietic tissues have shown that chromosome anomalies are present, but they are very variable and lack consistency. Furthermore, apart from Ph' no marker chromosome has so far been identified which could be considered to be a characteristic and specific component of the karyotype in a particular malignant condition of the haematopoietic system.

Marker chromosomes of similar morphology have been observed in *testicular tumours* (MARTINEAU, 1966; RIGBY, 1968) and in tumours of the *colon* (LUBS and KOTLER, 1967). One or more very long ("giant") acrocentric chromosomes in association with other abnormal chromosomes were encountered in 40 out of 63 malignancies analysed by ATKIN (1970). The incidence of these markers in three different tumour types is shown in Table 25.

A long acrocentric chromosome similar to that seen by ATKIN was also found in melanoma, and tumours of the breast, lung, colon, bladder and larynx (BENEDICT et al., 1968). In six patients with CML, lymphosarcoma, reticulum cell sarcoma and melanoma, a long acrocentric marker chromosome was described by GOH (1968). The presence of a similar chromosome in many diverse tumour types suggested to some investigators that this particular abnormal chromosome may represent a specific chromosomal change occuring during the carcinogenic process.

Minute *"chromatin bodies"* which probably represent centric chromosome fragments have been found in tumours of neural origin, (neuroblastoma, medulloblastoma, glial tumours); the number of such bodies varies in cells, in some more than 50 were counted (Cox et al., 1965).

Table 26. Clonal evolution of abnormal karyotypes in a trisomic leukaemic child
(LEJEUNE et al., 1963)

Number of chromosomes	Karyotype
47	Trisomy — 21
48	Trisomy — 21 + 1G
49	Trisomy — 21 + 2G
50	Trisomy — 21 + 2G + 1D
51	Trisomy — 21 + 2G + 2D
52	Trisomy — 21 + 2G + 2D + 1C
53	Trisomy — 21 + 2G + 2D + 2C
54	Trisomy — 21 + 2G + 2D + 2C + 1F
55	Trisomy — 21 + 2G + 2D + 2C + 2F
60	Trisomy — 21 + 2G + 2D + 2C + 2F + 1E + 3C + 1A

Another importance of marker chromosomes is that their presence in several cells indicates a common origin from one progenitor cell. The number of cells with the same marker may show great variation, depending on how much the proliferative capacity of the cell has been increased. In some tumours the proportion of cells with the marker may be very high. Thus WAKONIG-VAARTAJA (1962) observed a large metacentric chromosome in 99 per cent of cells in a carcinoma of the uterus; a similar finding was reported by ATKIN and BAKER (1966). In Ewing's sarcoma two marker chromosomes were found in 271 out of 272 metaphases analysed by PORTER et al. (1969). Marker chromosomes not only provide evidence that part or the whole population of malignant cells are derived from a common ancestor, but they also enable us to follow the evolution of further aberrations in chromosome constitution. The study of different karyotypes in a case of chronic myeloid leukaemia led FORD and CLARKE (1963) to suggest that the various karyotypes could represent closely related clones, all derived from a common ancestral cell, but the acquisition of supernumerary chromosomes altered the original chromosome pattern, conferring a selective advantage on the cell. In similar case of acute congenital leukaemia in a trisomic-21 mongol, LEJEUNE et al., (1963) carried out karyotypic analysis and demonstrated a continuous stepwise evolution of new chromosome patterns by successive acquisitions and duplications of extra chromosomes. Table 26 shows the nine stages in the pathway which resulted in the "evolution" of a karyotype with 60 chromosomes.

Further studies of chromosome constitution in leukaemic cells, particularly during the blastic crisis, confirmed this concept of clonal evolution of abnormal karyotypes (BERGER, 1965; DE GROUCHY et al. 1966). These studies revealed the pathways of clonal evolution which occurs in three stages: (1) the acquisition of extra chromosomes and occasionally duplication of the additional chromosomes; (2) loss of specific chromosomes; (3) structural rearrangements. The results of the three pathways may be present together, and these complex changes, both numerical and structural, make the karyotypic analysis very difficult. DE GROUCHY and co-workers (1968) analysed several cases of CML and observed all the various stages of clonal evolution; the general scheme of progressive changes are illustrated in Fig. 27.

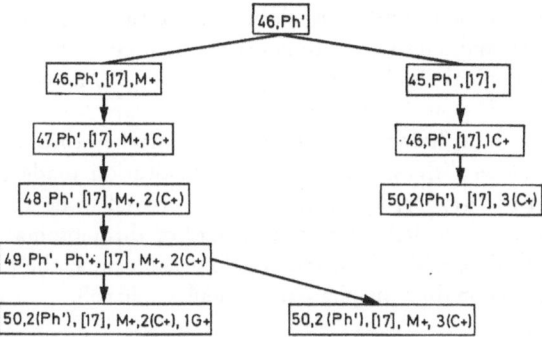

Fig. 27. Scheme showing three pathways of clonal evolution of leukaemic cells with 50 chromosomes; +sign indicates addition of supernumeraries, M⁺: marker chromosome; [17]: loss of chromosome 17 (After DE GROUCHY et al., 1968)

SPIERS and BAIKIE (1968 b) found similar stages of "cytogenetic evolution" during the acute transformation of CML, when extra chromosomes of the G, E and C groups were successively acquired by the 46-chromosome cells with Ph'; these steps were followed by duplication of the C group chromosomes. These findings and similar observations by other authors (PEDERSEN, 1971 and BAUKE, 1971) support the view of LEJEUNE et al. (1965) according to whom in CML undergoing blastic crisis the *"variant commun"* is a cell with Ph' in which the progressive changes affect mainly the chromosomes from group G, E and C. The acquisition of a supernumerary chromosome is commonly the first step in clonal evolution of aneuploidy, and is followed by duplication of the extra chromosome.

The occurence of such an event has been observed by FRACCARO et al. (1968) in a benign cystic adenoma of the ovary, the histological appearance of which indicated the onset of cancerous transformation. The analysis of 114 dividing cells revealed three basic karyotypes of cells with 46, 47 and 48 chromosomes. The increase of chromosome number from 46 to 47 and 48 was due to one and two extra C chromosomes; the frequency of the three classes of cells was 45, 18 and 5 per cent respectively. FRACCARO and his co-workers believe that in this particular cell population they "have witnessed the very beginning of an evolutionary process leading towards more pronounced aneuploidy and malignancy".

Summary

Structurally altered "marker" chromosomes, distinguishable from chromosomes in the normal human karyotype, have been observed in most tumours. The most remarkable marker is Ph' (Philadelphia chromosome), an abnormal chromosome 22 which has lost a large segment of its long arm. Ph' is associated with chronic myeloid leukaemia and is present in the cells of the haematopoietic tissue; it is the first, and so far the only, chromosomal anomaly which is a constant and specific feature of a particular malignant condition. The Ph' chromosome was found to be a very valuable marker for diagnosis and prognosis. The occurence of morphologically similar, abnormal chromosomes in a number of malignancies of a particular kind, has been reported by various investigators. Of interest are a very long acrocentric and another submetacentric chromosome, and it is claimed that they may be considered to be marker chromosomes characteristic of tumours of the lung, testis and colon. The claim is based on morphological similarity, though according to a recent study this is not necessarily evidence of "genetic" identity.

The presence of morphologically recognisable marker chromosomes in a group of cells with otherwise different chromosome constitution made possible the study of clonal evolution of karyotypic aberrations. Ph' proved to be a very useful marker for such studies, which revealed the various stages of chromosomal aberrations occuring during the "blastic crisis" of chronic myeloid leukaemia, the progressive changes indicating the increased malignant phase in the leukaemic cell.

Chapter 10

Chromosomes in Precancerous Lesions and in Tumour Development

Cytogenetical studies of human tumours have been carried out mainly on advanced stages of malignancies, it can therefore be argued that the chromosome anomalies observed are far removed from the primary events of the carcinogenic process, and should only be considered to be secondary effects of malignant transformation. If chromosome anomalies have a role in this process, the study of chromosome behaviour in precancerous lesions could be expected to provide relevant information. Such studies have been pioneered by Dr. A. I. SPRIGGS' Cytodiagnostic Unit at Oxford, who investigated chromosome abnormalities in carcinoma *in situ* and dysplasias of the uterine cervix, which are the most suitable lesions for such studies as about 40 per cent develop into invasive cancer.

The first report by SPRIGGS et al. (1962) on six cases of precancerous cervical lesions showed the chromosome number deviated from the diploid number in most of the dividing cells analysed. Clones of cells with marker chromosomes were observed in two cases, and in both other biopsy specimens taken from different regions showed "early micro-invasive foci", indicating that the lesion was progressing towards a more malignant stage. The second report from the same centre contains the findings obtained in nine cases diagnosed as dysplasia and carcinoma *in situ* (BODDINGTON et al., 1965). The data obtained provided further evidence that the chromosome number in cells of precancerous lesions is aneuploid, the cells being hyperdiploid and hypo-triploid; cells with hyper-tetraploid chromosome numbers showing more than one modal number were also found. Aneuploid cells with the same number of chromosomes were observed in several cases, indicating clonal proliferation of the chromosomally abnormal cells. Marker chromosomes were observed in most lesions. Though the number of dividing cells which could be analysed was small, the studies revealed that the epithelium of cervical lesions of incipient cancer contain aneuploid cells and that the range of variation in chromosome number was wide.

The findings of SPRIGGS and co-workers were corroborated by other investigators. WAKONIG-VAARTAJA and KIRKLAND (1965) drew attention to the fact that in dysplasias, variation in chromosome number is restricted around the diploid mode, while in carcinoma *in situ* the spread of chromosome variants is wide, and in one case they identified two modes; one was near-diploid and the other in the triploid-tetraploid range. In order to overcome the technical difficulties and to obtain larger numbers of dividing cells for chromosome analyses, RICHART and CORFMAN (1964) used tissue culture methods. Chromosome counts and karyotypes were prepared from biopsy samples of dysplasia and carcinoma *in situ* of the uterine cervix. The data obtained in five cases of pre-cancerous conditions is shown in Table 27.

In each case a diploid mode and "predominantly" normal karyotypes were found, in one case of dysplasia a marker chromosome was identified, similar to one described by BODDINGTON et al. In another series of nine cases studied using the same culturing method, similar data was obtained by RICHART and WILBANKS, (1966).

Table 27. Chromosome counts in cells of cervical lesions, cultured *in vitro*. (After RICHART and CORFMAN, 1964)

Histology	Number of Cells with Chromosome Count[a]				
	Hypo-Diploid	Diploid (Pseudo-)	Hyper-diploid	Hypo-triploid	Tetraploid (Appr.)
Mild Dysplasia	2	44	3	—	1
Moderate Dysplasia	4	45	—	—	1
Severe Dysplasia	5	43	1	—	1
Ca. *in situ*	3	42	—	1	4
Ca. *in situ* (microinvasion)	6	38	3	—	3
Total	20	212	7	1	10

[a] 50 cells were analysed in each case

Table 28. Chromosome constitution and range of variation in 97 cervical lesions (After AUERSPERG et al., 1967)

Histology	No. of lesions	Peri-diploid	Peri-triploid	Peri-tetraploid	Multiple modes
Dysplasia	36	80.5[a]	5.5	13.9	nil
Ca. *in situ*	61	19.6	13.1	45.9	21.3

[a] for purpose of comparison, the number indicates percentage

It is interesting to note that the incidence of aneuploid cells was 26 per cent, which is the same as these investigators found in control cultures of normal fibroblasts. In view of the contrary findings of others it is likely that either the cell population cultured *in vitro* was derived from normal epithelium, or that most of the aneuploid cancer cells failed to proliferate under *in vitro* conditions. The authors however, argue that by locating the exact position of the "cancerous" epithelium in cervical lesions, the few chromosomally abnormal cells are true neoplastic cells, and the heterogeneous cell population of invasive carcinomas are derived from them.

Data concerning the chromosomal status of the cell populations in precancerous lesions of the cervix published up to 1966, were surveyed by AUERSPERG et al. (1967), and are given in Table 28.

Comparison of the figures revealed significant differences between dysplasia and carcinoma *in situ*; the former lesions have a near-diploid, the latter a near-tetraploid mode. The range of variation in chromosome number is wide in carcinoma *in situ* and more than one modal number was observed in several cases. A large marker chromosome was also identified, and the authors interpreted it as one from group

A(probably chromosome 2) which had undergone pericentric inversion; this chromosome is referred to as the "*API-marker*" (so called because it is a group A pericentric inversion). The data from previous cytological studies of dysplasias, carcinoma *in situ* and invasive carcinomas which were obtained by direct squash techniques have also been analysed by JONES et al. (1968) and are given in Table 29.

The chromosome constitution in 73 per cent of dysplasias analysed is in the diploid range. The lower incidence of near-diploid modes in the other two lesions strongly suggest that the near-diploid cells in dysplasias are neoplastic and undergo further chromosomal changes; they are the source of the grossly aneuploid cells of

Table 29. Range of variation in modal chromosome number in 184 cases of cervical lesions
(After JONES et al., 1968)

Histology	No. of lesions analysed	Peri- diploid	Peri- triploid	Peri- tetraploid
Dysplasia	30[a]	73.3	10.0	16.6
Ca. *in-situ*	55[b]	47.2	21.8	30.9
Ca. cervix (invasive)	99	57.0	33.0	10.0

[a] in one patient three biopsy materials were analysed
[b] in one patient four biopsy materials were analysed

carcinoma *in situ* and invasive carcinoma. The authors argue that the presence of aneuploid cells (even those that are near-diploid) is strong evidence for considering the lesion to be "malignant". However, the diagnosis of a lesion as cancer on a chromosomal basis does not necessarily mean that the lesion will progress into the "invasive" stage. Instances are well known in cytopathology in which the appearance of exfoliated cells with characteristics highly suggestive of malignancy, failed to develop into clinical cancer.

A comparative study of the range of chromosomal variation in the three cervical lesions: dysplasias (4 cases), carcinoma *in situ* (22 cases) and invasive carcinoma (35 cases) was carried out by WAKONIG-VAARTAJA and HUGHES (1965) and HUGHES (1965). In order to analyse the distribution of chromosome numbers, the cell populations were grouped according to their ploidy levels. Data obtained by analysing 1,417 cells revealed differences in the chromosome patterns between the three kinds of lesions, (see Fig. 28).

The frequency of cells with chromosome constitution in the near-tetraploid range is much less in the invasive carcinoma than in carcinoma *in situ*. This shift in the frequencies of ploidy levels is due to a decrease in the number of "polyheteroploid" cells (with chromosome numbers between 69 and 103).

These findings raised the question: can the changes observed in chromosome pattern be related to the onset of invasion from the pre-invasive stage? This problem was investigated by CELLIER et al. (1970), who employed the method of WAKONIG-VAARTAJA and HUGHES to analyse the chromosome counts obtained from cervical lesions of 156 patients. In order to classify the lesions according to the number and type of ploidy, each carcinoma was described in terms of estimates of two parameters: the mean of chromosome counts and the variance from the mean. The material analysed comprised 4,134 cells, an average of 26 cells per case. Their data are in agreement with the work of WAKONIG-VAARTAJA and HUGHES, and show that the

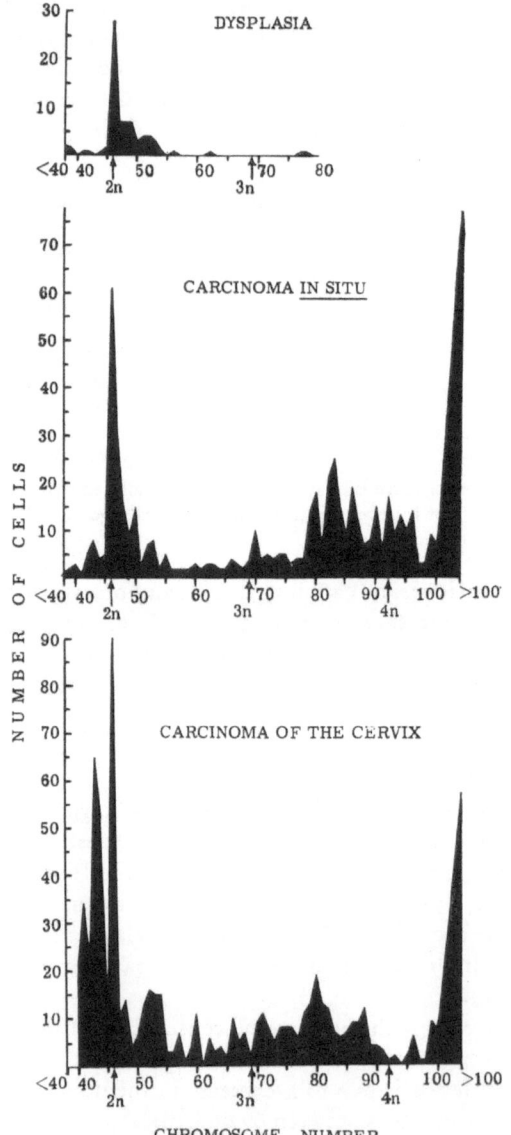

Fig. 28. The ploidy levels in cervical lesions (By courtesy of Dr. D. T. HUGHES)

onset of invasion is accompanied by a reduction in the number of ploidy classes. It seems that during the process of transition the range of variation in chromosome number became narrower than it was in carcinoma *in situ*.

The data obtained by these two groups of investigators suggest that from the wide range of chromosome variants present in carcinoma *in situ,* only a small group of aneuploid cells in a particular class (diploid or triploid) participate in progression towards invasiveness. It appears that cells with high chromosome numbers in the hyper-tetraploid range are either incapable of continued proliferation or are eliminated from the cell population. Mitotic abnormalities which occur frequently in the "polyheteroploid" cells may be responsible for their disappearance.

While the relatively low number of peri-tetraploid cells in the invasive carcinoma of the cervix appears to be a characteristic feature, the cytogenetic structure of invasive tumours at other sites differs from that of cervical carcinoma. Thus the predominant cell population of invasive carcinoma of the bladder is hypo-tetraploid (LAMB, 1967), and the invasive adeno-carcinomas of the colon have cell populations of high ploidy class (LUBS and KOTLER, 1967).

Chromosomes of benign and malignant lesions of the breast have been studied by TOEWS et al. (1968). Cystic mammary disease, a benign condition, has only cells with the normal chromosome constitution; *in situ* lobular carcinoma contained mostly diploid cells and a few showing aneuploidy. In the invasive breast tumours the triploid range was the most common mode. The ploidy level in breast tumours however, has little value in prognosis for it has been found that diploid tumours can invade and metastasize. The cytological data so far available for breast tumours seem to indicate that progression from a localized benign towards an invasive malignant stage is not always associated with gross numerical changes in chromosome constitution. The presence of structural chromosome aberrations in the cells (fragments, rearrangements, multiradial configurations, rings and morphologically distinct marker chromosomes) are more important in prognosis since high frequencies of chromosomal aberrations in the tumour have been found to be associated with a greater malignancy.

Adenomatous benign polyps of the colon very often show areas of "atypical" cells, forming glandular structures embedded in the regular pattern of the adenoma; these regions can be considered to represent incipient carcinoma *in situ,* which may overgrow the adenoma and progress into invasive carcinoma (ENTERLINE and ARVAN, 1967). The chromosome pattern of typical adenomas consists of pseudo-diploidy and hyperdiploidy. In adenomas with "atypical" regions the incidence of aneuploid cells is high, and the chromosomes of hyper-diploid cells exhibit structural aberrations resembling the chromosomal pattern of cells in the invasive carcinomas. One may therefore assume that the greater chromosomal disturbances in these particular areas of the benign adenoma is evidence of carcinogenic influences in action. In view of these findings it seems that in pathological lesions a high incidence of chromosomally abnormal cells, and a wide range of variation in aneuploidy, can indicate the lesion to be a precancerous condition which may progress towards the stage of invasive cancer.

In order to obtain information which could demonstrate an association between the type and frequency of chromosome aberrations and the onset of leukaemia, long term investigation of *preleukaemic conditions* has been carried out by NOWELL (1971). He studied such conditions in fifty-one patients who were followed for several years after chromosome studies of their bone marrow cells were made. No chromosome aberrations were found in patients with anaemia, leukocytosis, neutropenia and thrombocytopenia, and during the course of the investigation (which lasted many years) none developed leukaemia. Chromosomal anomalies were observed in the marrow of patients with myeloproliferative disorders which included polycythaemia vera and pancytopenia; in some such patients leukaemia developed within three months, while in others no leukaemia appeared during the years the patients were under observation. Four patients with no chromosome aberrations in their marrow cells developed leukaemia (one within 3 weeks of the chromosome study). NOWELL's investigation shows that a "preleukaemic" state may be present without chromosome aberrations and can develop into frank leukaemia. On the other hand, the presence of chromosome aberrations indicates an increased risk of leukaemia, but if however, the disease does not manifest itself within a few months of diagnosing the chromosome anomalies, the leukaemic risk remains the same as in comparable patients without chromosomal changes. In view of these later findings, the author revised the conclusion he had reached from previous studies, that individuals with "preleukaemic condition" who had in their bone marrow a clone of cells with chromosome abnormalities were very much more likely to develop leukaemia than those without chromosomal aberrations (NOWELL, 1965).

The data available from the cytological studies reviewed above, show that when chromosomally abnormal cells are present, progression from a precancerous state towards invasive cancer may be predicted. The cellular components of precancerous and cancerous tissue usually exhibit a variable spectrum of chromosomal aberrations, and they may reflect the degree of malignancy and histological structure of the tumour. LAMB (1967) undertook a cytological study on a series of transitional-cell carcinomas of the bladder and was able to relate variation in chromosome numbers with the degree of cellular differentiation and prognosis. His study covered 30 carcinomas of the bladder in various stages of differentiation and invasion. Tumours in the "well-differentiated" group were found to be characterized by diploid modal numbers with a narrow range of chromosome variation, while the less differentiated tumours had hypo-tetraploid modes and a greater range of variation in aneuploidy, (see Fig. 29 and 30).

The data obtained by LAMB demonstrate a correlation between chromosome ploidy and invasiveness in bladder carcinomas (see Fig. 31).

According to LAMB carcinomas with hypo-tetraploid modes have the worst prognosis, while those with near-diploid modes have the best prognosis.

Evaluation of possible clinical-cytogenetical correlation has also been attempted for other tumours. ATKIN (1964) made an assessment of the prognostic significance of chromosomal changes in carcinoma of the cervix. The data obtained by ATKIN seem to indicate that the well-differentiated squamous cell carcinomas of the cervix exhibit aneuploidy with a near-diploid mode and poor clinical prognosis, while tumours in the hyper-tetraploid range are less-differentiated yet show a relatively favourable prognosis and are comparatively less malignant. The situation is quite different in carcinomas of the corpus uteri; for those with high chromosome numbers, (estimated by micro-spectrophotometry and chromosome counts) the prognosis is significantly worse than for the majority of tumours which have near-diploid modes. ATKIN observed that the latter groups consist of well-differentiated tumours, while the poorly differentiated tumours had modes in the near-triploid or near-tetraploid region (ATKIN, 1970). It seems therefore, that the relationship between the pattern

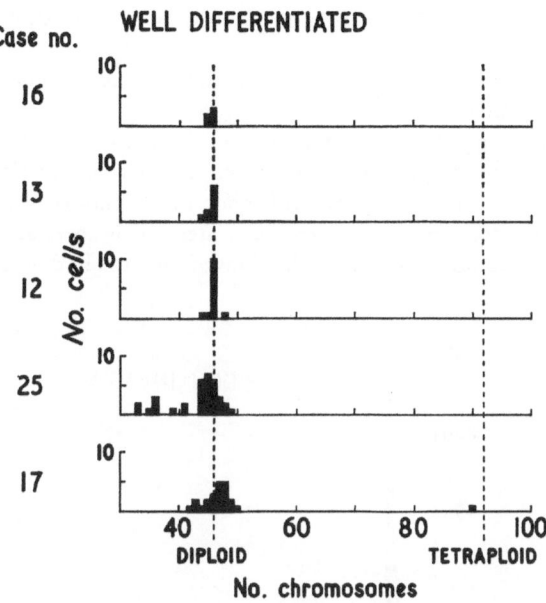

Fig. 29. The chromosome constitution in well-differentiated transitional-cell bladder carcinomas (By courtesy of Dr. D. LAMB)

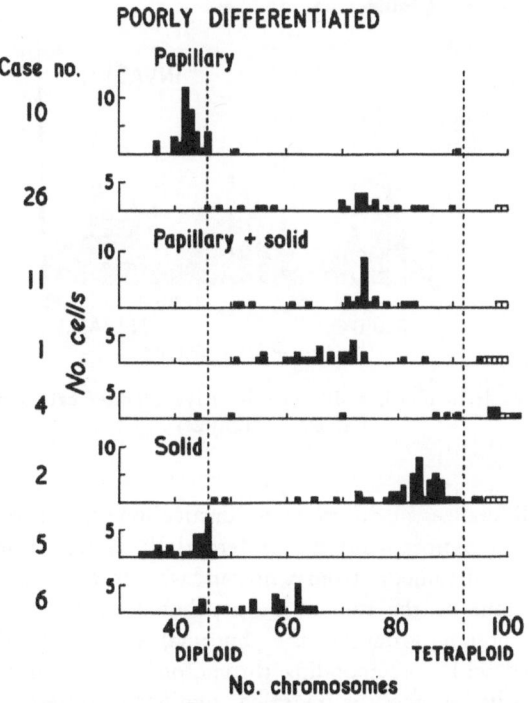

Fig. 30. Modal chromosome number and range of chromosomal variation in three histological
types of bladder carcinoma (By courtesy of Dr. D. LAMB)

of chromosomal variation, degree of differentiation and prognosis varies between tumours at different sites.

These examples suggest that correlation between histopathology, the pattern of chromosomal variation and prognosis does occur, but in a characteristic fashion for any given type of tumour; e. g. near-tetraploid mode in carcinoma of the cervix is correlated with good prognosis, in carcinoma of the uterus it is correlated with poor prognosis. One may ask: could the diverse behaviour of tumours be due to qualitative rather

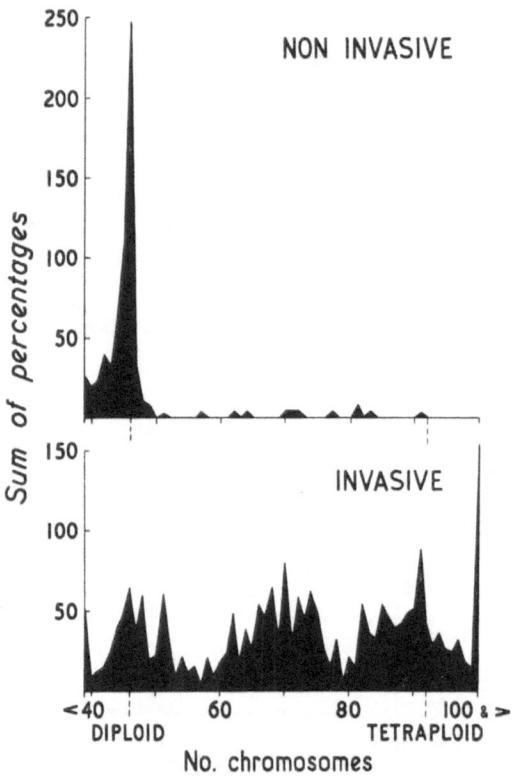

Fig. 31. The ploidy levels in non-invasive and invasive bladder carcinoma (By courtesy of Dr. D. T. HUGHES)

than quantitative differences in chromosome constitution? Are there certain chromosomes or groups of chromosomes which are preferentially increased or decreased during oncogenic progression of tumours from a non-invasive to an invasive stage? Can the characteristic behaviour of the tumour be attributed to the new constellation of chromosomes? Chromosome groups in the abnormal karyotypes of various tumours have been compared with corresponding chromosome classes of the normal human karyotype, and statistical analysis revealed significant differences. Thus STEENIS (1966) found that in a variety of tumours the chromosomes of groups D and G were under-represented, while chromosomes in group C were over-represented. A different karyotypic pattern was found by Wakonig-Vaartaja and Hughes (1967) who restricted their comparative analysis to carcinoma of the cervix and employed a more rigid statistical method; they observed chromosome losses in groups B and E as well as the changes in groups C, D and G reported by Steenis. These studies show that certain chromosome groups are more frequently affected than others during the conversion of a normal cell to a neoplastic one, but fail to explain the diverse behaviour of malignant cell populations on a chromosomal basis.

Summary

Cytological studies of precancerous lesions of the cervix demonstrated the presence of cells with aneuploid chromosome constitution. In the early stages of the development of the lesions (referred to as dysplasia), the deviation in chromosome number is restricted around the diploid mode, while in carcinoma *in situ* the range of deviation is wider, and occasionally more than one modal number could be identified. It seems that the progression of histological changes from dysplasia to carcinoma *in situ* is associated with greater chromosomal aberrations; in the latter, both the incidence of chromosomally abnormal cells and the degree of aneuploidy is greater than in dysplasias. Comparison of chromosome constitutions between carcinoma *in situ* and invasive carcinoma revealed a lower incidence of peri-tetraploid cells in the latter. In view of this observation, it is assumed that in the process of progression towards the invasive stage only diploid and triploid cells participate, the high-ploidy cells are eliminated through mitotic abnormalities. While the chromosome constitution in cervical lesions may be used as an aid to prognosis concerning the degree of malignancy, chromosomal alterations in precancerous lesions at other sites follow a different pattern, e. g. in the invasive stage of carcinoma of the bladder, the predominant cell type is hypo-tetraploid. The data so far available from studies on tumour development, indicate that the relationship between the pattern of chromosomal variation, degree of histological change and progression towards invasiveness, varies between tumours at different sites.

Chapter 11

Chromosomal Predisposition to Cancer

Cells with aneuploid chromosome numbers have been demonstrated in precancerous lesions, most of which are known to develop into invasive carcinomas. The question may therefore be asked: does the aberrant chromosome constitution favour the malignant transformation of cells?

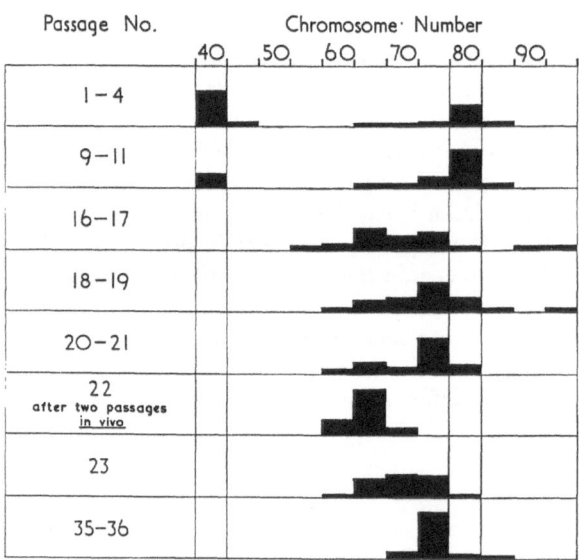

Fig. 32. Changes in chromosome number in an embryonic mouse skin culture; the cell population was malignant when tested *in vivo* at the 22nd passage (After LEVAN and BIESELE, 1958)

One of the best pieces of evidence for an aneuploid chromosome constitution having such a role is the observation of LEVAN and BIESELE (1958). These authors grew embryonic mouse skin *in vitro* and analysed the chromosome constitution of the cell populations of successive passages; their findings are shown in Fig. 32.

The histogram illustrates the changes in chromosome number observed in the cultures of the different passages. After the 21st. passage, the chromosomally grossly altered cell population was tested for carcinogenicity by subcutaneous grafting into mice, in which sarcoma subsequently developed. The malignant nature of the sarcoma was proved by transplantation into new hosts. The cytological analysis revealed the various stages in the transformation process; the first was a shift in the chromosome number from diploidy to tetraploidy, and by the 16th. passage no diploid cells were seen in the cultures. The range of variation in chromosome number stretched from hyper-diploidy to hyper-tetraploidy. The second stage was represented by a reduction in the number of chromosome variants, which occured in passage 20; after *in vivo* passage, the chromosome constitution of the cell population became hyper-triploid and had a narrower range of variation than was observed in previous passages. The most important events occured during the first four passages, when a very high incidence of mitotic abnormalities (chromosome bridges, non-disjunction, chromosome fragmentation, multipolar spindle) was observed in the proliferating cell population. The findings of these authors demonstrate that in this case chromosomal changes preceded malignant transformation, and strongly support the view that an abnormal chromosomal constitution favours the carcinogenic process.

A similar role for chromosomal anomalies is indicated by the experiment of YoSIDA et al. (1970). Syrian hamster embryonic cells were cultured *in vitro*, exposed to the carcinogen: nitroquinoline-oxide, and the chromosome constitution was examined in different stages of culturing. Altogether eleven cell lines were obtained showing "morphological" and chromosomal changes: four cell lines were predominantly composed of diploid or near-diploid cells; five had near-tetraploid modal numbers; two others were bimodal with near-diploid and near-tetraploid modes. The cell lines were tested for carcinogenicity by transplanting them into cheek pouches of adult hamsters or into subcutis sites of newborn animals. Amongst the "diploid" group, one cell line is of special interest; the majority of cells examined 37 days after treatment with the carcinogen had the normal diploid karyotype (44 chromosomes). When the cell line was tested for carcinogenicity in the animals, it produced a small nodule which regressed. The same cell line was analysed again a month later, the modal chromosome number was found to be 43, and the missing chromosome was identified as the small submetacentric chromosome 12 of the hamster karyotype. This cell line was again tested for carcinogenicity, and tumours were produced in which the range of variation in the number of chromosomes was between 43 and 47. When tested, the other cell lines with near-triploid and near-tetraploid modes all produced tumours.

The sequence of cytological events occuring in the liver of rats fed on p-dimethylamino-azobenzene has been analysed by GLÄSS (1960) and STICH (1963). Progression towards the development of malignant hepatoma is characterized by numerical changes in the chromosomes of liver cells, which occur well before the neoplastic process has been completed. Malignancy was tested by transplantation of liver tissue; tumours developed after a long latent period during which the diploid cells were replaced by cells with a near-tetraploid chromosome number. These aneuploid cells comprised about 55 per cent of the malignant cell population. Similar observations were made by the present author who studied the development of thymoma in C57Bl mice which had been given total body irradiation. Chromosomally abnormal cells appeared in the irradiated thymus well before the thymus lobes could be shown to be malignant through transplantability tests.

The findings of these experiments lend importance to the presence of chromosomally abnormal cells in precancerous lesions. It may be considered that the abnormal chromosome content in the cell represents the "chromosomal imbalance" which, according to BOVERI, is the underlying cause of neoplasia. Here it is relevant to describe the statistical approach taken by GOFMAN and associates, (1967) to investigate the validity of BOVERI's hypothesis. According to these investigators, the "imbalance" may be expressed by an "abnormal ratio of chromosomes of a particular type to chromosomes of another type, in contrast to the analogous ratio in the normal diploid cell". The sophisticated statistical analysis carried out by them, seemed to indicate that chromosome 16 in group E, is the most important component responsible for the "imbalance" of chromosomal constitution which characterizes the karyotypes of malignant cells in established cell lines. Further study in which human cancers (effusions) were analysed, yielded similar results, demonstrating both absolute and relative chromosomal "imbalance" which centred on the excess of chromosome 16. The author's claim that chromosome 16 in the human karyotype has a special and decisive role in cancerization of cells is based on computerized data obtained from studies on only seven cell lines and two cancerous effusions, and its validity has yet to be proved.

In order to assess the proportional representation of chromosome types in malignant and normal cells, MULDAL and co-workers (1971) employed a similar computer method. Their study showed a significant gain in group C and losses in groups D and G. According to these authors, the excess in group C comes from isochromosomes and translocations, particularly those between chromosomes of the acrocentric groups (D and G). Translocations of this type are also most common in human karyotypes. As the acrocentric chromosomes with satellites contain the special "nucleolar organizer" segment, translocations involving these chromosomes may lead to a progressive loss of such regions. Early cytochemical and cytological studies of cancer cells drew attention to the possible role of the nucleolus in the initiation of malignant cell behaviour (KOLLER, 1943). If this chromosomal impairment is relevant to cancer, individuals carrying such translocations would have an increased tendency to develop tumours. Should future investigation show that carriers of D/G translocations have a higher incidence of cancer than those without them, the finding of MULDAL and co-workers will be of great importance in detecting persons with a predisposition to cancer.

The increased incidence of cancer in persons with a constitutional chromosomal anomaly (described in Chapter 2), is further evidence that chromosomal predisposition to cancer does exist. The best example of such an association between chromosomal abnormality and malignant disease is Down's syndrome and leukaemia. In 1958, STEWART and co-workers reported that of 677 children dying of leukaemia, 18 were "mongols"; the incidence being tweny times higher than in normals (STEWART et al., 1958). Mongolism is associated with trisomy of chromosome 21, and is a constitutional chromosome anomaly. Patients with other syndromes caused by chromosomal aberrations, and who developed cancers, have been reported in the literature, and the question has been asked: is there a relationship between an abnormal chromosome constitution and susceptibility to the development of malignant disease? Is the frequency of constitutional chromosome aberrations in cancer patients higher than in normal persons? Table 30 shows the incidence of different types of cancer observed in 1,149 patients with abnormal karyotypes.

Of the eight patients with cancer, six had autosomal and two sex chromosomal abnormalities. However, though the incidence of autosomal anomalies (0.5 per cent) is higher than in controls (0.15 per cent), the figures are too small to attribute much significance to them at present (HARNDEN et al., 1969).

Table 30. Incidence and type of malignancy in 1,149 persons with constitutional chromosome aberrations[a]. (HARNDEN et al., 1969)

Types of malignancy	Chromosome constitution
Lymphosarcoma	45, D/D translocation
Ca. lung	46, Pericentric inversion C
C. mouth	47, one supernumerary chromosome
Ca. cervix	47, XXX
Ca. breast	45, D/D translocation
Ca. breast	46/47 mosaic
Lymphosarcoma	46, Pericentric inversion Y
Ca. ovary	46, 2/C translocation

[a] A further and more recent survey of 1,919 cancer patients revealed only 12 additional constitutional chromosome aberrations, which suggests that the incidence of cancer in such individuals is not higher than in the general population. (Personal communication by Professor D. G. HARNDEN).

A group of Russian oncologists analysed the chromosome constitution in 100 patients with various types of leukaemia, and found four with chromosomal aberrations; one with a balanced D/D translocation and three others in which there was an enlarged A1 chromosome, large Y and an altered D chromosome respectively; the three latter anomalies were interpreted as normal variants of the human karyotype (PRIGOGINA et al., 1970). In another case of chronic myelocytic leukaemia, chromosome studies revealed that the patient was a D/D translocation carrier (ENGEL et al., 1965). Malignancies have also been observed in patients with Klinefelter's syndrome (FRAUMENI and MILLER, 1967), and instances reported in which sex chromosome mosaicism was associated with tumours of the gonads; it appears that persons with abnormal gonadal differentiation (true hermaphrodites) are prone to develop gonadoblastomas, (FERRIER et al., 1967).

Cases in which a particular chromosome anomaly is present in several members of a family, some of whom developed malignant disease, are of special interest. Such a case has been reported by GUNZ et al. (1962). The abnormal chromosome referred to as Ch' was believed to be chromosome 21 of group G, it had lost all or the greater part of its short arm. The abnormal chromosome is shown in Fig. 33, and the pedigree of this family living in Christchurch (New Zealand) is given in Fig. 34.

When the family was first investigated, two members (nos. 4 and 6) had the Ch' chromosome and lymphocytic leukaemia, three others (nos. 3, 7 and 15) had Ch' without leukaemia. More recently the same Cytogenetic Unit reported the development of chronic lymphocytic leukaemia in a third sibling (no. 3) who was a carrier

of Ch'. Cytological analysis of peripheral blood lymphocytes was also carried out
in five other members of the family (10, 11, 14, 17 and 18) who were found to be
non-carriers. Using ^{3}H-thymidine autoradiography the authors identified the Ch'
chromosome to be the same as Ph'; i. e. chromosome 22. In view of these findings,

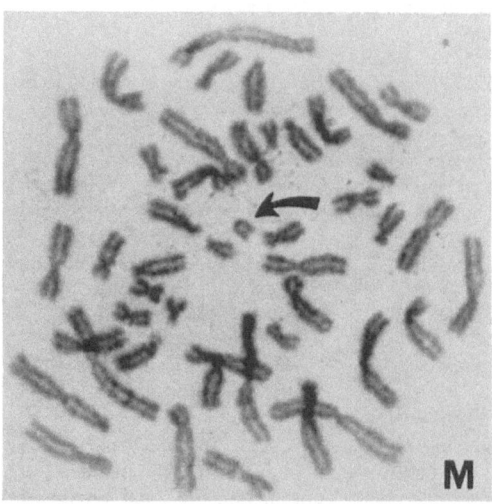

Fig. 33. Karyotype showing Ch' chromosome in a male (M) leukaemic member of the New
Zealand family (By courtesy of Dr. P. H. FITZGERALD)

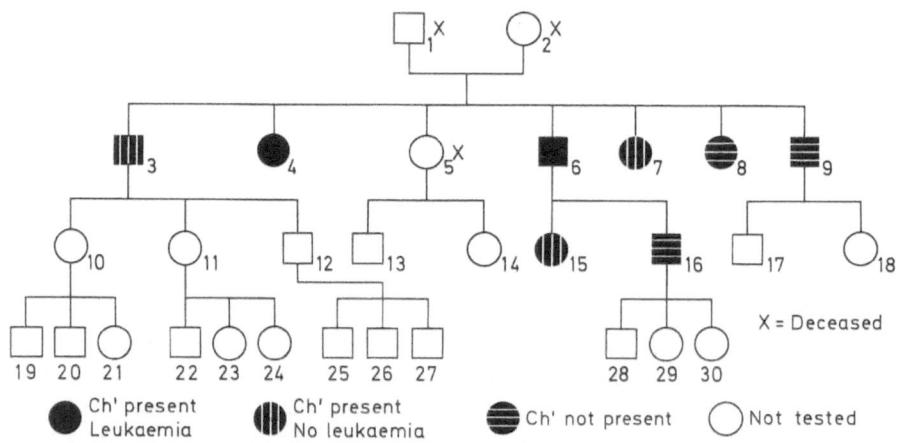

Fig. 34. Family pedigree showing the association of the defective chromosome (Ch') with
leukaemia (After GUNZ et al., 1962)

Ch' chromosome may be considered to be a predisposing factor to leukaemia in this
family (FITZGERALD and HAMER, 1969). In another family with a high incidence
of cancer, chromosome studies revealed an abnormally long chromosome 1 or 2 of
group A; it was present in five members of this family: three had carcinoma of the

breast, the fourth squamous cell carcinoma of the skin and the fifth was a carrier of the abnormal chromosome without cancer, (MERZ et al., 1968). Though few reports concerning the association of constitutional chromosome aberrations with cancer have been made, they are nevertheless important for the clinician, who should be aware of the possibility that chromosome aberrations may predispose to malignant disease. Predisposition or susceptibility to cancer may also be investigated on a cellular basis by the technique of TODARO et al. (1966). These investigators found that the Simian virus (SV40) transforms cells grown *in vitro*, and confers on them the following malignant properties: (1) loss of contact inhibition (the cells grow in colonies instead of monolayers); (2) the presence of T-antigen and (3) an ability to produce tumours (tested by inoculation of the cells into susceptible hosts). (See Chapter 12.)

The fraction of cells transformed can be used to measure the sensitivity of cells to transformation. Through this method TODARO and his associates (1966, 1967) have demonstrated that fibroblasts from the skin of patients with Down's syndrome and Fanconi's aplastic anaemia exhibit increased sensitivity to transformation by SV40; both conditions are known to predispose to leukaemia and other malignancies (SWIFT and HIRSCHHORN, 1966).

Table 31. Frequency of cell transformation *in vitro* by SV-40. (TODARO et al., 1966)

Source of cells	Number of transformed colonies[a]
Controls (7)	1.6 — 5.1
Fanconi's anaemia	
Homozygotes:	
AM	79.7± 18.1
JV	41.1 ± 12.1
Heterozygotes:	
TM	20.1 ± 3.2
CV	28.2 ± 8.7

[a] 10,000 cells plated

Fanconi's anaemia is an inherited disorder, conditioned by an autosomal recessive gene. The disease is characterized by chromosome anomalies, aplastic anaemia and congenital malformations affecting the skeletal system. The former consist of chromosome and chromatid breaks and rearrangements in the somatic cells of the affected individuals. Bloom's syndrome is another disease with an increased expectancy for the development of leukaemia and other malignancies; it is probably under simple genetic control, and is characterized by low birth-weight, stunted growth and skin sensitivity to sunlight. It has been shown that there is a tendency to chromosomal breakage and rearrangement in cells of such patients, when cultured *in vitro* (SAWITSKY et al., 1966). These findings led to the hypothesis that fibroblast sensitivity to viral transformation will identify persons at high risk of leukaemia and perhaps of other malignant conditions (MILLER and TODARO, 1969).

Table 31 shows the frequency of cell transformation in four members of a family; two were homozygotes having inherited from both parents the genes predisposing to the disease. In this family the number of transformed colonies was 50 times higher than in cells of normal persons. A higher frequency of transformation by SV40 in the fibroblasts from a lung cancer patient with Klinefelter's syndrome and XY/XXY mosaicism has been reported by MUKERJEE et al. (1970). Fibroblasts from skeletal muscle were grown *in vitro*, and chromosome analysis revealed two cell types present: one with XXY and the other with XY sex chromosome complements. As controls, fibroblast cultures of skeletal muscle tissue from two men and two women were used. Table 32 shows the transformation frequency of the fibroblasts by SV40.

The data indicate that cells from the patient with Klinefelter's syndrome have a higher frequency of transformation than cells from normal controls, and that the XXY cell strain is more sensitive to transformation than the XY cell strain of the same patient. By identifying the Barr-bodies present, the frequencies of cells with XXY or XY chromosome constitution in the lung tumour were found to be 65 and 35 per cent respectively; the frequency of XXY cells is significantly in excess of the frequency expected according to those observed in the patient's leukocyte cultures.

Table 32. Transformation frequency of fibroblasts by SV40 in controls and patient with Klinefelter's syndrome. (After MUKERJEE et al., 1971)

Cell-strains	Karyotypes	Transformation frequency per 10^4 cells	No. of foci per 8×15^5 cells
Control males	$44 + XY$	2.7 ± 0.10	199
Control females	$44 + XX$	3.0 ± 0.15	243
Cell-strains in patient	$\{ 44 \pm XY$	9.7 ± 0.30	780
	$\{ 44 \pm XXY$	28.5 ± 4.30	2282

The finding strongly suggests that the abnormal chromosome constitution conferred on the cells a greater susceptibility for malignant transformation.

The relationship between an abnormal chromosome constitution and susceptibility to transformation has been investigated by PAYNE and SCHMICKEL (1971). Fibroblasts from four different sources were exposed to the virus SV40, and the presence of T-antigen in the cells was taken as an indication of transformation; the antigen was detected by the indirect immunofluorescence technique using serum from hamsters bearing SV40-induced tumours. Table 33 shows the relative susceptibilities of different cell strains to SV40 T-antigen induction.

The trisomic cells of Down's syndrome exhibited greater susceptibility than triploid cells; since the former cells (2N + 1) have a more "imbalanced" chromosome constitution than that of triploid cells (3N), it can be inferred that the greater this imbalance, the more increased the cellular susceptibility to transformation becomes. The findings of these investigators, together with the studies of cell behaviour in Fanconi's anaemia and Bloom's syndrome, suggest that chromosome anomalies might be one of the signals of abnormal cellular conditions, which can predispose to malignant transformation. It might be possible therefore, to use chromosome anomalies which occur in the cells of persons exposed to environmental agents as indicators of the carcinogenic hazards of these agents. Chromosome analysis of individuals in occupations which are known to contain such hazards have already been made, and revealed a significantly higher frequency of chromosomal aberrations in the peripheral blood cells of exposed persons than in controls. Two examples may be described to illustrate the possible significance of chromosomal aberrations.

Studies on luminous-dial painters demonstrated a higher incidence of cells with chromosome aberrations than in a random sample of controls, and showed a consistent gradient of increasing chromosome abnormality with increase in the body content of radium (BOYD et al., 1966). Chromosomal studies were carried out on individuals exposed to benzene, which is known to be toxic to the haematopoietic-system, and is now becoming recognised as a leukaemogen. FORNI and MOREO (1967) followed a case of "benzene anaemia" which developed into acute myeloblastic leukaemia after a long latent period. A high rate of chromosomal aberration was found in the cultured peripheral blood lymphocytes during the period of severe anaemia which preceded the onset of leukaemia. These instances strongly suggest that chromosomal aberrations occuring in the cells of peripheral blood, might be used as indicators of carcinogenic hazards.

Table 33. Susceptibility to SV 40 transformation of fibroblasts with various chromosome constitution (After PAYNE and SCHMICKEL, 1971)

Group	No. of estimations	Percentage of cells with T-antigen (5×10^4 cells/ml were exposed to SV 40)
Normal-control	7 (3)[a]	8.8
Triploid	4 (1)	7.8
Trisomic	4 (2)	18.1
Fanconi	2 (1)	39.8

[a] number in brackets indicates number of patients donating skin fibroblasts for culturing.

Nowadays the natural environment of man is undergoing rapid changes; the great variety of chemical substances and drugs introduced into industry, food manufacture and medicine, bring new problems in their wake, and it has been found that not infrequently the use of such agents is linked with unspecified dangers to health. Cytological analysis of cells for chromosomal effects could indicate the carcinogenic potentiality of these agents.

Summary

Evidence that aberrant chromosome constitution predisposes cells to malignant transformation has been obtained through *in vitro* and *in vivo* experiments. It was found that the deviation from the normal diploid constitution is brought about by mitotic anomalies which indicate intracellular metabolic disturbances, assumed to be a preliminary stage in the carcinogenic process. The result is a numerical alteration, i. e. chromosomal "imbalance" in the karyotype, which may further enhance the transforming process. The assumption that cells with chromosomal anomalies become susceptible to neoplastic transformation, is supported by the association of particular malignancies with constitutional chromosome aberrations (Down's, Klinefelter's syndromes etc.). Another example of chromosomal predisposition is the familial incidence of chromosomal aberration and development of leukaemia in the carrier of the anomaly. The high frequency of malignant disease in persons with genetically determined chromosomal instability (Fanconi's and Bloom's syndromes), is another evidence suggesting that chromosomal anomalies may act in cells as predisposing factor towards malignancy. The cytological studies of these phenomena can lead to the application of the *in vitro* method of TODARO for identifying persons with a high risk of cancer.

Chapter 12

Chromosomes and Viral Oncogenesis

The first tumour virus was discovered more than sixty years ago by the Italian physician CIUFFO (1907). He found that cell-free filtrate from human papilloma or wart material produced warts when injected under the skin of volunteers. In the following year ELLERMAN and BANG (1908) transmitted erythroblastic leukaemia in chickens using cell-free filtrates. Their observations were confirmed, and the properties of the virus subsequently investigated by ROUS (1910) and others. For many years the fowl was the only animal in which virus-induced tumours could be demonstrated, and was therefore considered to be a very special case. The real interest in studying oncogenic viruses started with the report that viruses produced tumours in mammals. SHOPE (1932) described virus-induced papillomas in rabbits, BITTNER (1936) demonstrated that mammary tumours in mice harbour a virus, and GROSS (1951) discovered the very important mouse leukaemia virus. There are now over 25 different viruses known to cause tumourous growths in at least one species of animal (RAPP and BUTEL, 1970).

During the past decade, with the discovery of new viruses (polyoma, Simian-40, adeno-virus 12, Epstein-Barr virus) much research has been carried out and a great amount of knowledge accumulated concerning the interaction between viruses and mammalian cells. Improved methods enabled easy culturing of mammalian cells *in vitro*, and the emergence of molecular biology provided the tools for investigating the basic mechanism of malignant transformation of cells. The present chapter summarises the findings of recent research, their relevance to cancer in man, and the possible role of chromosomes in viral oncogenesis.

Viruses are sub-cellular microorganisms dependent for their existence and multiplication on the host cell which they infect. The genetic information determining the properties of the virus is coded in their nucleic acid, by which tumour viruses are classified into two groups: RNA- and DNA-viruses. Table 34 gives examples of the two kinds of tumour viruses.

Some tumour viruses are transmitted from parent to offspring (vertical transmission), and may also spread by contact (horizontal transmission). Mammary tumour virus in mice is transmitted through the milk, leukaemia virus through the placenta. The fowl leukaemia virus can be passed from generation to generation through the egg, but it can also spread by contact. It has been demonstrated that the virus present does not always produce a tumour in the animal (silent infection), the animal is only the carrier and transmits the virus to the progeny in which it may produce tumours. This is the case in the fowl leukaemia virus and the mammary tumour virus in mice.

Cytological studies of tumours associated or induced by RNA oncogenic viruses indicate that the malignant behaviour of infected cells is under the direct control of the virus, and that the host cell's own genetic apparatus, as represented by its chromosomes, has an indirect role. Chromosomal analysis of 91 primary tumours induced in mice by injection of Rous sarcoma virus has shown that the great majority of sarcomas were diploid; the deviation from the normal karyotpye was small, and specific chromosomal aberrations were absent (MARK, 1967). In 42 tumours induced by the same virus in Chinese hamsters, the most common stemline was composed of diploid cells, deviation from the diploid number consisted in the addition of one, two or three extra chromosomes. Karyotyping revealed 28 different patterns, and a progressive decrease of diploid cells in the cell population of older tumours (KATO, 1968). Similar findings have been reported concerning the chromosome constitution of tumours induced by Molony's, Friend's and Rauscher's murine leukaemia viruses.

Table 34. Oncogenic viruses

RNA-viruses	DNA-viruses
Rous sarcoma	Papilloma viruses[a]
Fowl leukaemia	(human wart, rabbit etc.)
Mouse leukaemia group	Polyoma[a]
Mouse mammary tumour virus	Simian vacuolating virus (SV40)[a]
Mouse sarcoma virus	Adenoviruses (12, 18)

[a] Papilloma, polyoma and SV40 viruses are referred to as the PAPOVA-group, (Pa = papilloma; Po = polyoma and Va = vacuolating virus)

The possible role of chromosomal aberrations in the aetiology of a virus-induced leukaemia has been investigated by RICH et al. (1964). The virus used by these authors induced thymic lymphoma within 50 days of inoculation, and the various stages of leukaemogenesis could be followed. Cytological studies have shown that the cell population of the histological lesion (termed "lymphoma-in-situ" and limited to one of the parallel thymic lobes) was normal; the appearance of aneuploid cells coincided with an invasion of the opposite healthy thymic lobe. With the dissemination of the proliferating lymphoma to spleen, liver and peripheral nodes, the frequency of chromosomally abnormal cells progressively increased. The sparcity of aneuploidy in pre- and early leukaemia, and the high incidence of aneuploid cells in the disseminated lymphoma suggests that the chromosome changes represent one of the consequences of neoplastic transformation.

During the studies of mouse leukaemia a new virus: *polyoma* was discovered (STEWART et al., 1958). This virus can give rise to a great variety of tumours in many mammalian species (mice, rats, hamsters, rabbits, guinea pigs etc.). Polyoma is a DNA virus and can be isolated not only from leukaemic tissue but from normal tissues of wild mice. The virus can be maintained in cells grown *in vitro,* and its presence in an animal can be detected by serological methods. Under natural conditions polyoma only very occasionally produces tumours in adult animals, because the infected host defence mechanism eliminates the virus or virus-carrying cell. Tumours can be induced when the virus is injected into newborn animals in which the immune mechanism is not fully developed.

The injection of cell-free extracts from tumours or other tissues into newborn animals (usually hamsters), became an important procedure in cancer research. During the extensive campaign of polio vaccination in the late 1950's, it was discovered that the vaccine derived from kidney cell cultures of the green African monkey, contained the *Simian vacuolating virus* (SV40) which is a natural infection in this particular species of monkey. By injecting the vaccine and its virus contaminant into newborn hamsters, tumours were produced, (EDDY et al., 1961). This finding was of great importance since man is susceptible to SV40 infection and it was known that millions of people were already exposed to the virus before the danger was recognised. In the United States studies are in progress to detect a possible increase in the incidence of malignant disease in people who received the particular polio vaccine known to have been contaminated with SV40.

In the same year that the oncogenic property of SV40 was revealed, TRENTIN and co-workers (1962) tested a large number of adeno-viruses which cause infection in early childhood, and are responsible for epidemics of respiratory diseases in man. In the first test, *adeno-virus type 12* was found to produce tumours in newborn hamsters, in successive tests the tumour-producing activity of other adeno-viruses was also established. Both viruses: SV40 and Ad-12 are DNA viruses and have many properties in common; these viruses were found to be very suitable to study the process of malignant transformation of mammalian cells *in vitro*.

The ability of oncogenic viruses to transform cells grown *in vitro* made possible a study of the sequence of events which result in malignant cell behaviour. It was soon discovered that 6—10 hours after infection with papova viruses, a new antigen appears in the cell; it is localised in the nucleus of cells infected with polyoma and SV40; in Ad-12 infected cells it is also present in the cytoplasm. This antigen is called the *T-antigen* and can easily be demonstrated by the usual immunological techniques: complement fixation and fluorescent antibody test. By applying these methods it was found that the T-antigen of a given virus is identical whether the infected cell is of hamster, rat or human origin; the T-antigen is specific for the virus, indicating that the genetic information coding for the antigen is derived from the viral genome.

The next stage in the process of transformation is the *stimulation of DNA synthesis* in the cell. It was found that 10—12 hours after infection with polyoma or SV40, the activities of enzymes involved in the biosynthesis of DNA e. g. thymidine kinase, are increased to a value about 3—10 times higher than in non-infected cells. Those viruses which are known to be oncogenic have the property of stimulating DNA synthesis in the host cell, whereas on infection by other non-oncogenic viruses e. g. vaccinia, rabies etc. DNA synthesis was inhibited. It has been found that the fixation of the transformed state as a heritable property of the cell requires at least one cell division after infection; transformation does not occur in non-dividing cell populations.

The effects of virus infection on chromosomes of the host cell have been investigated through *in vitro* and *in vivo* systems. Many studies have been carried out and the findings indicate that the types of chromosome injuries associated with viral infection are very similar to those induced by X-rays and chemical agents. It was found that viral replication is necessary to induce chromosomal aberrations which may occur in the very early stages of viral infection. Extensive chromosomal damage (breaks, dicentrics) in cells infected with SV40, coincides with loss of contact inhibition which is closely related to tumourigenicity *in vivo*. "Pulverization" of chromosomes is a frequent event seen in cells infected with measles, Sendai, adeno-viruses and virus vaccine against Yellow fever (MOORHEAD, 1970). Several chromosome studies of tumours induced by Shope rabbit papilloma virus, polyoma and SV40 have been carried out and diploid or near-diploid chromosome constitutions were found in the majority of primary tumours. The development in rabbits of benign virus-induced papillomas towards invasive carcinoma has been followed in 25 primary epidermoid tumours by McMICHAEL et al. (1963); it was observed that the incidence and extent of chromosomal aberrations increased with time, and that the stemlines of the similar tumours were karyotypically all different. Primary tumours induced by polyoma in mice have been found to have diploid stemlines; after transplantation into new hosts the chromosome constitution of the tumour underwent changes, and according to HELLSTRÖM and co-workers (1963) often conferred a selective advantage on cells with an aneuploid chromosome number. The findings of cytological studies indicate that chromosomal anomalies seen in virus-induced tumours are secondary effects.

There are two important aspects which concern the presence of the oncogenic virus in the cell: (1) the number of viral genomes required for transformation and maintenance of the transformed state, and (2) the region within the viral genome which is reponsible for transformation. By using RNA and DNA hybridization methods it was estimated that less than 20 viral genomes were present in polyoma transformed cells. For transformation by SV40, one viral genome was found to be sufficient; on further evidence however, it was found that only half of the SV40 genome was involved in transformation. Later studies revealed that in polyoma transformed cells, not more than half of the viral genome was operating to maintain the transformed state. Experiments which aimed to recover polyoma from the transformed cells have so far failed, but proved successful when SV40 transformed cells were tested, yielding the complete SV40 viral genome.

Cells transformed by RNA and DNA viruses do not yield infectious virus particles (except under very specific conditions). Despite failing to recover complete viruses from transformed cells, there is evidence to show that the viral genome is present. The strongest proof is the presence of T-antigen in the transformed cells and tumours induced by the virus; it seems that this antigen is permanently associated with the transformed cell. As regards the location of the viral genome in the transformed cells, it was postulated that the viral genome may be stably integrated into the host's own chromosomes. To test the *"integration"* hypothesis, somatic hybrid cells which lose most or all of the chromosomes of one parental type, have been used. Fusion of cells yielding "hybrid cells" was first reported by BARSKI and co-workers (1960), who observed that when two lines of mouse cells, differing in chromosome constitution, were cultured together *in vitro*, a new cell type eventually appeared which contained within a single cell the chromosome sets of both parental cells. Hybridization of somatic cells of various kinds and of different species became an important method for the study of somatic cell genetics, including inborn errors of metabolism in humans. The discovery by WEISS and GREEN (1969) of the rapid elimination of human chromosomes from human-mouse hybrid cells made the method applicable for testing the "integration" hypothesis. In the experiments reported by WEISS (1970) SV40 transformed human cells were used in combination with various non-transformed mouse cells. The hybrid cells produced were isolated in a pure culture, karyotyped periodically and tested for the presence of SV40-induced T-antigen as an indicator for the presence of the SV40 genome. The analysis revealed that the number of human chromosomes in the hybrid cells declined with progressive cultivation, occuring most rapidly between the twentieth and fiftieth generation. Fig. 35 shows the decrease in the mean number of human chromosomes over more than 150 cell generations.

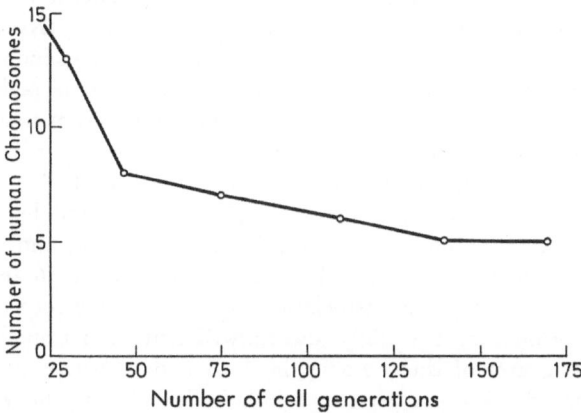

Fig. 35. Loss of human chromosomes from mouse x human hybrid clone; the most rapid loss occured between the 20th and 50th generation (After WEISS, 1970)

When the culture was tested for the presence of T-antigen, T-antigen-negative cells were found after 50 generations, and on isolation and karyotyping it was found that 90—97 per cent of the human chromosomes were lost in these cells. This finding suggests that the viral genome must be associated with the human chromosomes and that more than one chromosome acts as a carrier of the viral genome, the integration of which is stable. By hybridization of two mouse cell-lines with different karyotypes, MARIN and LITTLEFIELD (1968) observed the same effect with polyoma virus. These results strongly support the hypothesis of chromosomal integration of the viral genomes in the transformed cells.

Attempts have been made to identify specific effects which would indicate the "hot spots" of viral integration in the chromosome. Secondary constrictions representing achromatic gaps in particular regions of human chromosomes are the sites which are occasionally affected by viral infection. It has been reported that these specialized chromosome regions (many of them acting as nucleolar organizers) became attenuated, broken or despiralized in cells infected with various viruses. Cytological studies of cell lines derived from patients with Burkitt's lymphoma or infectious mononucleosis have revealed lesions in these chromosome regions. In both conditions, the presence of a Herpes-type virus has been demonstrated; the virus is referred to as the Epstein-Barr virus (EBV), first observed in a Burkitt cell line established by EPSTEIN et al. (1964). EBV is a DNA virus and *direct* evidence has been obtained by ZUR HAUSEN and co-workers (1970) for its regular presence in cells of Burkitt lymphoma and anaplastic nasopharyngeal carcinoma. By using a test system which involves DNA — DNA hybridization and tritiated thymidine labelling these investigators found that DNA extracted from EB virus, annealed with DNA derived from biopsies of Burkitt lymphoma and nasopharyngeal carcinoma, indicating the integration of the viral genome into the host cell's DNA. The possible number of the viral genomes present in the cells was estimated to be between one and twenty-six. Cytological analysis of lymphocyte cultures established from patients with the disease has shown that 5—45 per cent of the cells had one or two chromosomes in group C (possibly chromosome 10) which exhibited a subterminal secondary constriction or gap in the long arm, never seen in normal cells (KOHN et al., 1967; DIEHL et al., 1968). It has been suggested that the lesion was induced by the EB-virus and may reflect a specific activation of this chromosome region which has a role in cell proliferation. Other chromosome studies of EBV-positive cell lines however, either failed to show the presence of the "C chromosome marker" or have shown it in extremely low frequencies (MACEK et al., 1971). A critical study has been carried out by HUANG and co-workers (1970) on 16 cell lines, derived from patients with Burkitt's lymphoma or infectious mononucleosis, and they demonstrated the presence of the C-marker in only three lines out of the 16 analysed. According to them there is no apparent association between the presence of EB-virus and the C-chromosome marker. The study also showed that the terminal or subterminal regions in the long arm of chromosomes in A, B and C groups accumulated more lesions than other chromosome regions, which indicated that the virus can induce chromosome injuries. Non-random damage to chromosomes of human embryo kidney cells and fibroblasts have been observed after infection with Ad-12. The lesion induced was similar to that found in EBV-infected lymphoblasts, but in the former case it was located in the long arm of chromosome 17 of group E (McDOUGALL, 1970). It is interesting to note that the other adeno-viruses (type 2, 5, 7 and 18) produced only random damage to human chromosomes of cells cultured *in vitro*.

Virus-transformed cells, under certain conditions, can produce a high frequency of variants in which the characteristics of transformation (loss of growth control *in vitro;* tumourigenicity *in vivo*) have again been suppressed, yet such cells retained the viral genome. RABINOWITZ and SACHS (1970) investigated the cause of "reversion" in polyoma-transformed hamster embryo cells, and found that in the revertants, the chromosome number was much higher than in transformed cells. In view of this finding the authors put forward a hypothesis according to which "the expression or suppression of the characteristics of transformed cells depends on a balance between factors responsible for their expression (E) or suppression (S)". These factors are localised in certain chromosomes and are in balance in normal cells; addition of an extra chromosome carrying factor E upsets the balance and results in loss of growth control. On the other hand, the addition of an extra chromosome containing the S factor would cause reversion of the transformed cell into a cell which regained growth control. The chromosomes carrying E and S factors were identified by analysing the karyotypes of revertant hamster cells isolated from transformed cell populations exhibiting different degrees of transformed properties (HITO-

TSUMACHI et al., 1971). Using cell-hybridization techniques POLLACK et al (1970) provided evidence which seems to favour the hypothesis of RABINOWITZ und SACHS.

It is now well documented that DNA oncogenic viruses persist in transformed cells and are transmitted to progeny cells by the chromosomes into which the viral genome became incorporated. HUEBNER and TODARO (1969) surveyed the many reports concerning the evidence of viral aetiology of particular tumours in birds and mammals and suggested that in most, if not all vertebrates special viruses are present which play a role in the development of tumours; the unique property of this group of viruses is that the viral information can be transmitted from an animal to its progeny, and from cells to progeny cells, as a repressed viral genome (oncogene). According to the *"oncogene hypothesis"* the occurence of the majority of cancers is a natural biological event determined by spontaneous or induced activation or de-repression of the endogeneous specific viral genome which is incorporated into the host's chromosomal DNA. Polyoma, SV40, adeno-viruses (all DNA-oncogenic viruses) can be classified as "oncogenes" satisfying the requirements postulated by HUEBNER and TODARO. The difficulty arises as regards the RNA-viruses (Rous-sarcoma, murine-leukaemia, mammary tumour virus etc.). The question is: how can the genetic information of an RNA oncogenic virus be incorporated into the host cell chromosomal DNA?

Recent studies using methods of molecular biology revealed a mechanism which allows for such an event. It was discovered that RNA tumour viruses have the ability to make DNA with the help of a special enzyme: RNA-DNA polymerase. The enzyme is the product of the virus, and enables the RNA virus to transcribe the genetic information into DNA which, in this form, can be incorporated into the host cell DNA, with the help of two other enzymes: endonuclease and ligase. The incorporated virus is referred to as the "provirus" (TEMIN and MIZUTANI, 1970). This finding has been confirmed by other investigators, and according to them the RNA-dependent DNA-polymerase activity in a cell may indicate that the genetic information of the RNA oncogenic virus required for the transformation and maintenance of the transformed state, is present in the host DNA.

Following this important discovery, human leukaemic cells were analysed to see whether the RNA-DNA polymerase enzyme was present or not. According to a recent report the enzyme was detected in the extracts of human leukaemic cells; this finding implies that leukaemia in man might have a viral aetiology, and furthermore it offers a new way for detecting cancer at a far earlier stage of its development than is possible with present methods. The chemotherapeutic aspect of the discovery is stressed by GALLO and co-workers (1971) who succeeded in inhibiting the activity of this particular polymerase enzyme by the drug rifampicin. These investigators suggest that more effective drugs could be produced to selectively attack tumour cells *via* this mechanism. Their argument is valid if the production of DNA from RNA template is restricted only to cancer cells. According to more recent information however, RNA-dependent DNA polymerase enzyme has been identified in extracts of non-cancerous cells; DNA polymerase which can copy RNA-DNA has been found by SCOLNICK and co-workers (1971) in normal mouse and human cells, and has similar properties to those of the mouse leukaemia virus enzyme. Two other viruses were found which have enzyme activities similar to those of the RNA-containing tumour viruses. One is the syncytium forming "foamy" virus, a

common contaminant in monkey kidney cell cultures which causes giant multinucleate cells, the other is the "Visna" virus which is responsible for the progressive
neurological disease in sheep. These particular viruses have not yet been tested for
oncogenic properties.

Despite this setback, TEMIN's discovery remains a very valuable contribution to
molecular biology, for it shows that the genetic information which was postulated
by CRICK to be transcribed only from DNA to RNA can be reversed, it also gives
support to the oncogene hypothesis proposed by Huebner, and provides a mechanism by which RNA-containing viruses can become latent in mammalian cells.
AARONSON and TODARO (1970) found that the RNA sarcoma virus originating in two
different species (avian and murine) were able not only to grow in, but also to transform *in vitro* systems of human cells from diverse origins. This finding increases
the possibility that these or similar agents, may on occasion cross species barriers
and cause tumours in man.

Summary

Oncogenic viruses can transform the cells they infect, into malignant cells. There
are now about 25 such viruses known, and their number is still increasing. The genetic information which determines the properties of these viruses is coded in the
RNA or DNA molecule. Chromosomal analysis of primary tumours and leukaemias
induced by oncogenic viruses, has shown that the great majority of these malignancies are diploid, and if there is a deviation from the diploid chromosome constitution in the infected and transformed cell, it is very slight, but can undergo very
drastic numerical and structural alterations after several passages. The ability of oncogenic viruses to transform cells *in vitro*, made possible the identification of the various stages of the "transforming process". A virus specific T-antigen appears in the infected cell, in which DNA synthesis is stimulated. Though the infected cell does not
yield virus particles, there is evidence to show that the virus genome is present, being
integrated into the DNA of the host cells own chromosomes. The integration of RNA
viruses is negotiated by the RNA-DNA-polymerase enzyme, which has been identified
in both malignant and normal cells. The oncogene-hypothesis of Huebner suggests that
the majority of cancers are the product of spontaneous or induced activation of an
endogeneous specific viral genome present in the host's chromosomal DNA. Further
important progress can be expected from the intensive research studies now begun.

Chapter 13

Chromosomes and the Treatment of Cancer

The aim of cancer therapy is to destroy all malignant cells with proliferative capacity. By removing the cancerous growth surgery hopes to achieve this aim. When the malignancy is beyond the scope of surgery, the clinicians have the choice of radiation or administering chemical agents in order to bring about a cure or palliation. The purpose of the present chapter is to describe the effects produced in malignant cells by radiation and particular chemical agents, and to discuss their relevance to cancer therapy.

(1) *Radiotherapy* can claim considerable success due to the spectacular progress it made during the past 30 years. The introduction of new and powerful sources of radiation resulted in greater accuracy of treatment, higher depth doses and more uniform energy absorption, and these improvements led many clinicians to believe that a correspondingly large increase in the cure rate of cancer would be achieved. Though progress has been made, it is now admitted that the outcome of radiation treatment of tumours depends not on the precision of the physical parameters, but on the interactions of physical and biological factors. The present author made a systematic study of the biological factors which play an important role in the response of tumour cells and tissue to the following ionizing radiations: X-rays, radium, cobalt-60 and radioactive gold (^{198}Au); the results of these studies are reviewed below.

The effects produced by radiation on the cancer cell are of two kinds: temporary and permanent. The *temporary effects* consist of suppression of mitosis, stickiness of chromosomes, abnormal spindle formation, metaphase clumping of chromosomes; altogether these may be referred to as "physiological effects", amongst them the suppression of mitosis is the most important. The duration and time of onset of mitosis depends on the dose and may also be affected by the dose rate. The same radiation dose in different tumours produces different effects as regards the onset and length of mitotic free period. Morphological and biochemical evidence indicate that radiation interfers with DNA synthesis in the cell, and as a result mitosis is delayed. Another temporary effect of radiation is stickiness of chromosomes, the intensity of which is determined by the dose, in some cells it may cause the clumping together of metaphase chromosomes. The injuries referred to as "physiological effects" of radiation can result in death of the cells, but the number of cells thus destroyed is too small to be a significant factor in arresting the growth of tumours.

The *permanent effects* induced in malignant cells by radiation follow the same course as those observed in normal cells of experimental plant and animal material. These effects become visible in dividing cells several hours after exposure to radiation, and consist of various types of injuries to the chromosomes, the most obvious of which is a break in the chromosome strand, the distal segment usually appearing in post-metaphase stages as an acentric fragment. Dicentric chromosomes are the result of radiation-induced breaks in two chromosomes, followed by fusion of the centric parts; they can be identified during ana- and telophase when they form a double bridge between the two poles. In experimental material with few, large chromosomes these abnormalities can easily be recognised in the metaphase stage and have been used for quantitative analysis; in tumour cells however, it is difficult to identify and classify the various chromosomal injuries, owing to the small size and large number of chromosomes. Hence the quantitative and qualitative analysis of radiation effects have been restricted to the post-metaphase stages, in which acentric fragments and chromosome bridges could be easily observed and counted. Some acentric fragments may escape observation when entangled with the other chromosomes, consequently the number counted should be realized to be an underestimate. Both types of injury have serious consequences and they are usually lethal to the cell. There are various kinds of evidence to show that loss of genetic material from the cell nucleus impairs the metabolic pathways which are necessary for maintaining the proliferative capacity of the cell.

The development and consequence of the various chromosomal effects induced by radiation in tumour cells has been studied in biopsy material obtained from a large number of carcinomas of the skin and cervix (KOLLER and SMITHERS, 1946).

Figs. 36 a, b, c, and d show chromosomal effects in three tumour cells, 24—72 hours after irradiation with 100, 300 and 1,500 rads; the fourth cell which was

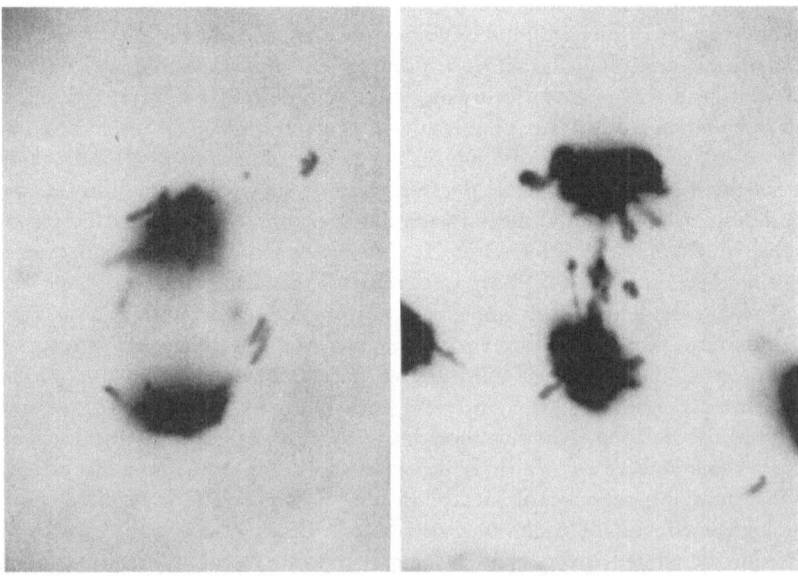

Fig 36a   Fig. 36b

Fig. 36. Radiation-induced chromosome injuries in human tumour cells after: a) 100 rads; b) 300 rads; c) 1,500 rads; d) 500 rads; the latter cell contains several micronuclei, formed by acentric chromosome fragments

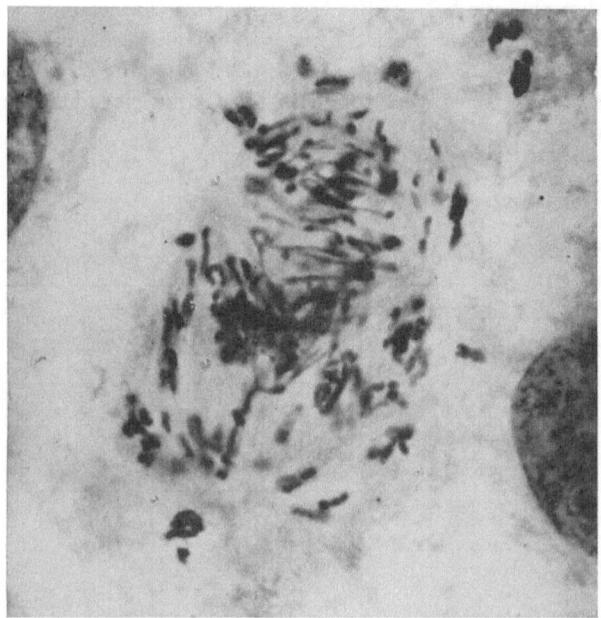

Fig. 36 c

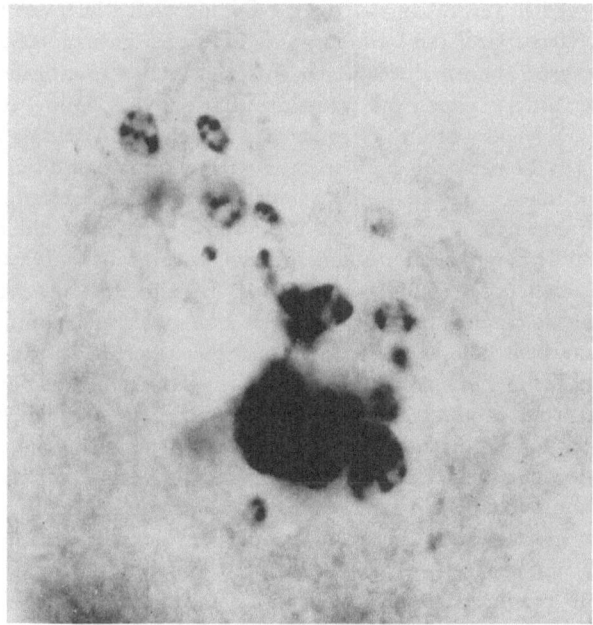

Fig. 36 d

irradiated with 500 rads contained several micronuclei in the cytoplasm. It was also observed that the number of dividing cells with chromosome injuries increased with the radiation dose; thus the frequencies of abnormal anaphases was 8, 14 and 27 per cent after 100, 300 and 1,500 rads respectively, (the data is an average estimate). Significant differences were found in the frequencies of abnormally dividing cells in different tumours which were exposed to the same radiation dose. Data obtained by analysing the chromosomal effects in three carcinomas of the skin are shown in Table 35.

Table 35. Radiation induced cellular damage in three tumours

Site	Percentage of injured cells	Percentage of cells with chromosome fragments									
		0	1	2	3	4	5	6	7	8	9—11
Cheek	13.5	86.5	0.5	3.0	3.5	4.5	1.4	0.5	—	—	—
Cheek	17.5	83.0	1.5	1.0	2.0	2.5	4.5	2.0	1.5	0.5	1.0—1.5
Forehead	8.5[a]	90.5	2.5	2.0	3.5	0.5	—	—	—	—	—

[a] 8 hours later the percentage increased to 12.0.
[In each case 200 dividing cells were analysed 24 hours after treatment with 300 rads]

The skin tumours were of the same histological type, located at similar sites and were of the same dimension, yet their response to the same radiation dose was different. Similar variations in radiation sensitivity of cells of different tumours have been observed in several instances; the finding well illustrates the difficulty of radiotherapists, who expect the same response after the same radiation dose is given.

The frequency of abnormal anaphases in serial biopsy specimens taken from the same tumour at different intervals after irradiation, was found to decrease with time. In one case 24 hours after 300 rads, the frequency of dividing cells with acentric fragments was 12 per cent, and no cells with chromosome injuries were seen in biopsy specimens taken from the same tumour 72 hours after radiation. This example of the declining effect of a dose of 300 rads, shows that it should have been much higher in order to destroy a greater number of cells with proliferative capacity. The administration of high doses (6,000—7,000 rads) to tumours, however, is associated with the risk of destroying cells of normal tissues which surround the tumour or form the tumour bed. The integrity and healthy state of these tissues have been found to be a *conditio sine qua non* for controlling the malignant growth by radiotherapy. Apart from producing chromosomal injuries in an increasing number of dividing cells, the high radiation dose also evokes a reaction in the connective tissue of stroma and tumour bed. The development and importance of this reaction have been followed and evaluated in serial biopsy specimens taken from carcinoma of the skin and cervix, after exposure to various radiation doses. It consists of the infiltration of various types of cells of the lymphoid series into the area surrounding the tumour, and into the intercellular spaces within the tumour itself. The polymorphonuclear cells and macrophages act as scavanger cells — and participate effectively in the healing process, which should follow the destruction of tumour tissue. The two events are illustrated in Fig. 37 a and b.

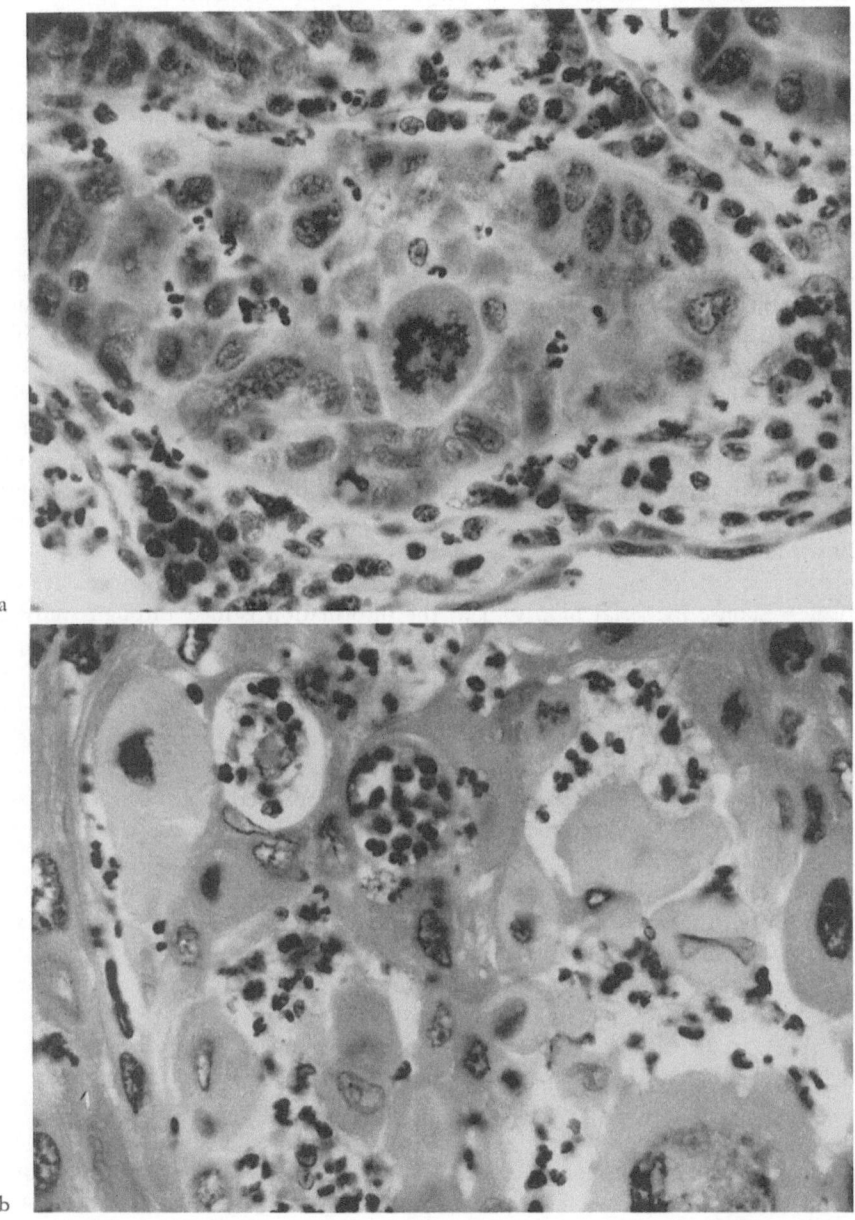

Fig. 37. Radiation-induced tissue-reaction: a) aggregation of reticulo-endothelial cells in the connective tissue surrounding the tumour; infiltration of leukocytes into the tumour. One tumour cell in mitosis contains injured chromosomes; b) infiltration of polymorphonuclear leucocytes and macrophages between and into degenerating tumour cells

A more detailed discussion concerning the nature of this tissue response to radiation in which the host's immune system plays an important role, is outside the scope of this book, and has already been described by the author in another publication under the title of "Biological Basis of Radiotherapy" (KOLLER, 1959). In view of the important role of the reaction of normal tissue and particularly the part cell components of the reticulo-endothelial system play in the dynamic process of radiation response of tumours, the principles derived from studies on isolated cells grown *in vitro*, though they are valuable, can in practice only be used by radiotherapists as vague suggestions when applying radiation to tumours in patients.

The "high" radiation dose required for therapy is administered by dividing it into smaller fractions. The time interval between successive radiation treatments and the size of the fractionated dose administered at each treatment are the two most important variables by which the cellular and tissue-reaction can be controlled. The time of delivery of successive radiation doses should coincide with the reappearance of dividing cells, a high percentage of which should have chromosomal injuries. Cytological analysis of biopsy material can give the information necessary to obtain a satisfactory response. In my experience, when treatment was controlled in this way, the growth of the tumour was not only arrested but also destroyed with doses considerably lower than those usually employed by radiotherapists. One such example is illustrated in Fig. 38.

In the treatment of most deep-seated tumours it is rarely possible to analyse cell and tissue response by serial biopsy. Yet, the information gained through study of the cellular response to various treatment schedules in accessible tumours has helped to design an experimental system of dose-fractionation which was tried out on tumours usually regarded as being radio-resistant (osteogenic sarcoma, spindle-cell fibrosarcoma, and chondrosarcoma). The treatment consisted in variations of increasing doses at increasing intervals (KOLLER and SMITHERS, 1946).

Fractionation of the radiation dose *in space* is another method by which the tissue reaction in tumour bed and stroma can be regulated. The method consists of using a lead shield with perforations of various sizes through which the radiation dose is administered (see Fig. 39). It was found that the tissue reaction was favourably affected by the presence of "protected" areas evenly distributed throughout the tumour and stroma (JOLLES and KOLLER, 1950 and 1953).

The importance of biological factors in tumour therapy has been realized and attempts have been made to increase cell sensitivity to radiation by various means. One of the most promising methods is the increase of oxygen supply to the tumour. It has been demonstrated in experiments that radiation-induced chromosome injuries are oxygen-dependent: the higher the oxygen concentration within the cell, the greater the chromosome injury. Much research has been devoted to the oxygen-effect on biological systems, and the therapeutic implications have been well presented by GRAY and his associates (1953). Histopathological analysis demonstrated that anoxic regions, usually the central areas in tumours (the source of recurrence), are radio-resistant (THOMLINSON, 1967). The principles based on experimental studies of oxygen effects on cell sensitivity have been applied to the radiotherapy of tumours, yet the therapeutic value of this method has yet to be shown. Perhaps the cause of failure experienced in practice lies in the fact that oxygen is known to have a dual role in the radiation survival of cells. It has been observed by LITTBRAND

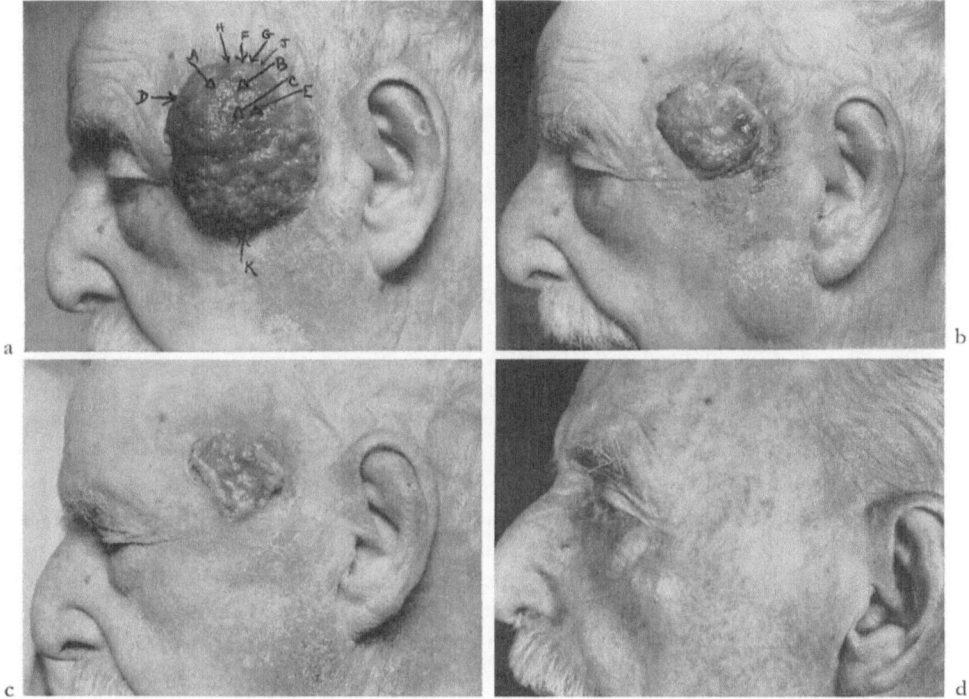

Fig. 38. Radiation response of a squamous cell carcinoma; a) before treatment, showing the sites of nine successive biopsies; b) seven days after completion of treatment (total radiation dose: 2,700 rads given over 19 days); c) fourteen days and d) nine months after treatment, showing no scarring at the radiated area (By courtesy of Professor Sir D. W. Smithers)

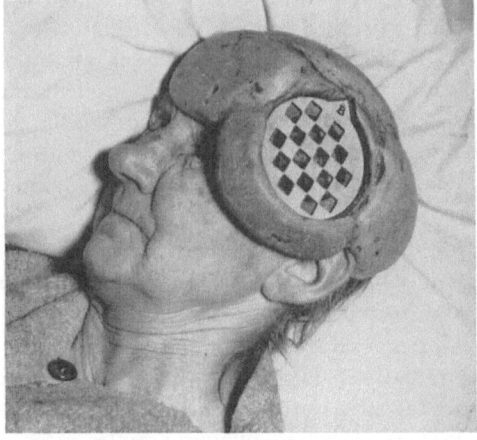

Fig. 39. Applicator used for fractionating of radiation dose in space (By courtesy of Dr. B. Jolles)

and RÉVÉSZ (1969) that oxygen sensitizes cells to radiation injury (chromosome breaks), but it also protects cells by permitting oxidative metabolism, which provides energy for the repair process of healing the breaks in the chromosomal DNA.

The study of chromosomal injuries has shown that treatment of tumours by radiation is not just a simple problem of geometry and applied physics, it is a complex process in which there must be a balance between biological probabilities and physical certainties. This view has been expressed recently by Dr. R. C. TUDWAY in his Presidential Address to the British Institute of Radiology in 1971. If progress is to be made, a better understanding of the biological basis of radiation injuries to cells and tissues is essential. Some of the problems which need to be clarified by radiobiological studies are: the sensitivity of hypoxic and oxygenated cells, the effect of radiation induced mitotic delay in tissues and the nature and mechanism responsible for recovery of cells between treatments. The investigation of the chromosomal basis of radiation injury and cell destruction carried out by myself and others was directed towards this aim.

(2) *Chemotherapy* is applied when the tumour is unsuitable for radiotherapy owing either to a widespread dissemination in the body e. g. leukaemias, or to a failure of the malignancy to respond to radiation. Many new types of chemical agents have become available since the Second World War, amongst them the alkylating agents form an important class. The first such agent to be administered to patients with cancer was the nitrogen mustard (methyl-*bis*-(β-chloroethyl)amine hydrochloride). The discovery of this group of agents is associated with the wartime study of the biological effects of the vesicant poison gas: sulphur mustard ($\beta\beta'$-dichlorodiethylsulphide), a nucleotoxic poison. The present author analysed the direct effect of this agent on the chromosomes of the plant *Tradescantia* and found that it damaged the chromosomes causing the death of the cell (KOLLER, 1947 b; see Fig. 40 a and 40 b).

Similar excessive chromosome injury has been observed in tumour cells of human effusions (see Fig. 40 c).

Since 1945 a large series of chemical substances have been synthesised in the Chester Beatty Research Institute (London), all of which show a common property in biological activity. The events resulting in growth inhibition of tumours in animals by alkylating agents have been studied by the present author, who found that the arrest of cancerous growth was due to injuries both to the chromosomes and to the mitotic apparatus of dividing cells. Fig. 41 a, b, c, d, e and f show the various types of chromosomal injuries in tumour cells, following administration of different doses of an alkylating agent.

Biochemical research indicates that nitrogen mustard acts by cross-linking the two polynucleotide strands of the DNA at the guanine base, resulting in breakage of the chromosome strand (BROOKES and LAWLEY, 1963).

The chromosome injuries produced by alkylating agents are very similar to those produced by ionizing radiations, hence these substances are referred to as "radiomimetic" agents. Besides the strictly radiomimetic effects, another kind of cytological disturbance has also been observed in tumour samples after the administration of alkylating agents. Amongst these effects superfragmentation of chromosomes and clumping of the injured chromosomes into several pycnotic bodies are the most common; these effects may be referred to as cytotoxic injuries; they occur about 72 hrs after treatment.

Comparison of the cytological effects produced by different alkylating agents revealed a direct relationship between the number of injured cells in the tumour and

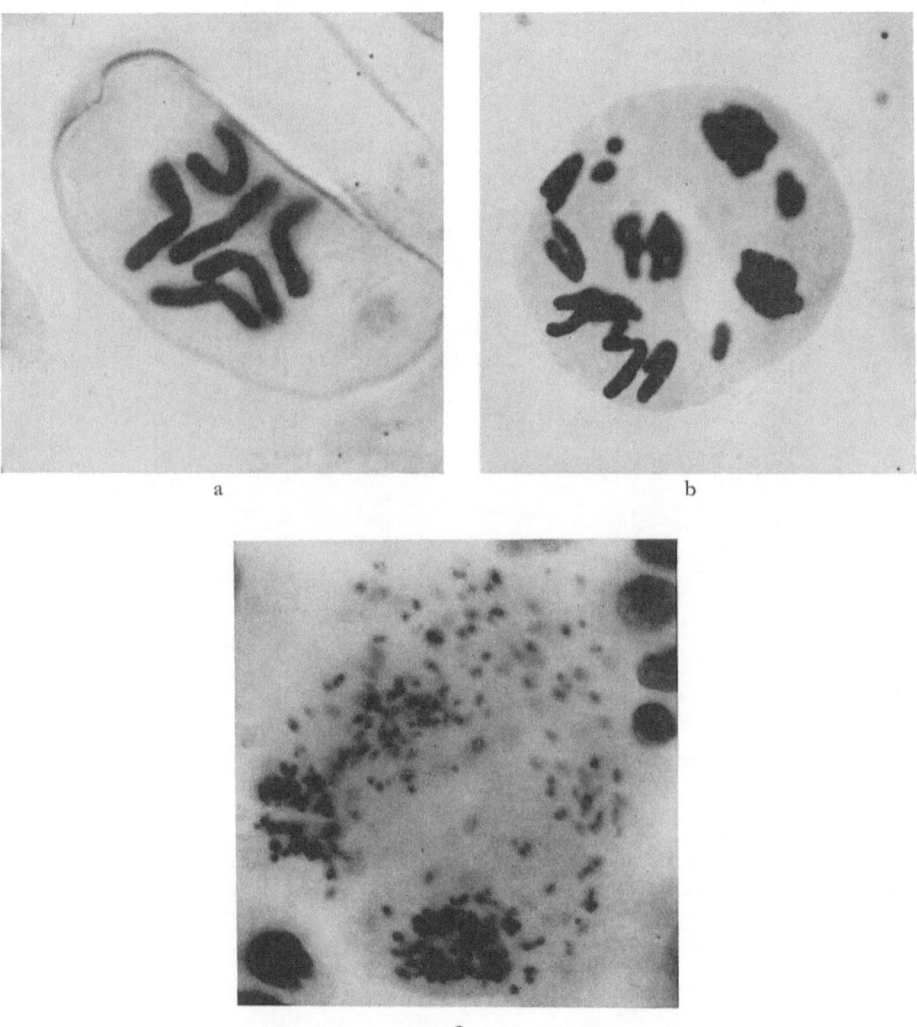

Fig. 40. Chromosome injuries induced in the cells of *Tradescantia*, exposed to sulphur mustard aerosol: a) before and b) after exposure; c) chromosome injuries in a tumour cell of human effusion, exposed to sulphur mustard *in vitro*

the extent of growth inhibition. Most of the alkylating agents produce cell injuries not only in neoplastic cells but also in cells of normal tissues e. g. bone marrow, intestine, testis etc. One member of the aliphatic sulphonic acid esters produced a particularly depressant effect on the circulating neutrophils of the rat (HADDOW

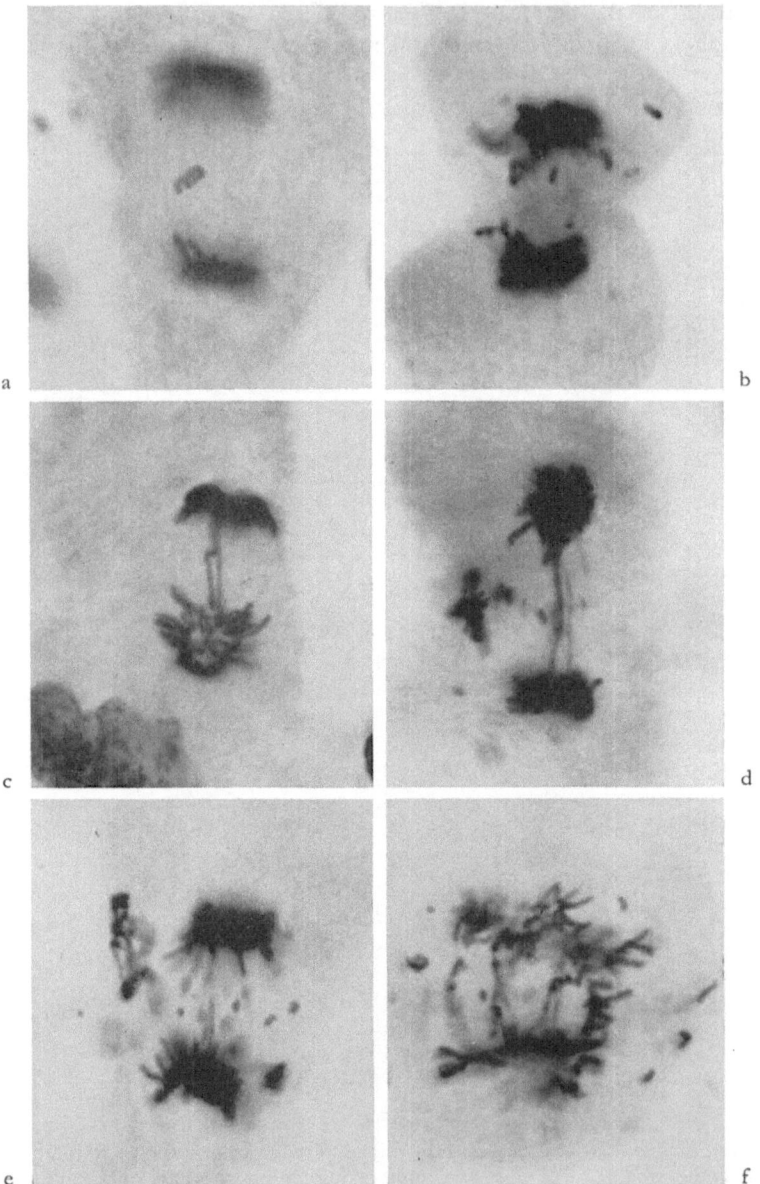

Fig. 41. Chromosome injuries in cells of Walker-256 carcinoma of the rat, induced by various doses of a nitrogen mustard derivative: a) 1 mg/kg dose i. p. 24 hrs after treatment; b) 1 mg/kg, i. p. 48 hrs after treatment; c) 1.5 mg/kg i. p. 24 hrs after treatment; d) same dose, 48 hrs after treatment; e) same dose, 56 hrs after treatment; f) same dose, 76 hrs after treatment

and Timmis, 1953). Cytological study disclosed that the maturation and release of granulocytes into the circulation was delayed, and the polymorphonuclear leukocytes had undergone degeneration. The *selective action* of this particular drug on blood cells of the granulocytic series led to its introduction into the therapy of myeloid leukaemia under the name of Myleran (Busulphan). The case of Myleran and Chlorambucil (another alkylating agent with selective action), illustrate that their therapeutic value in leukaemia is not wholly due to their radiomimetic properties. The rationale of chemotherapy is the selective killing of cancer cells by agents that interfere with cell division. X-rays, nitrogen mustard, imuran, cytoxan, vincaleukoblastine, amethopterin, D-actinomycin etc. are all effective to a variable degree against leukaemias and a few solid tumours, on account of their

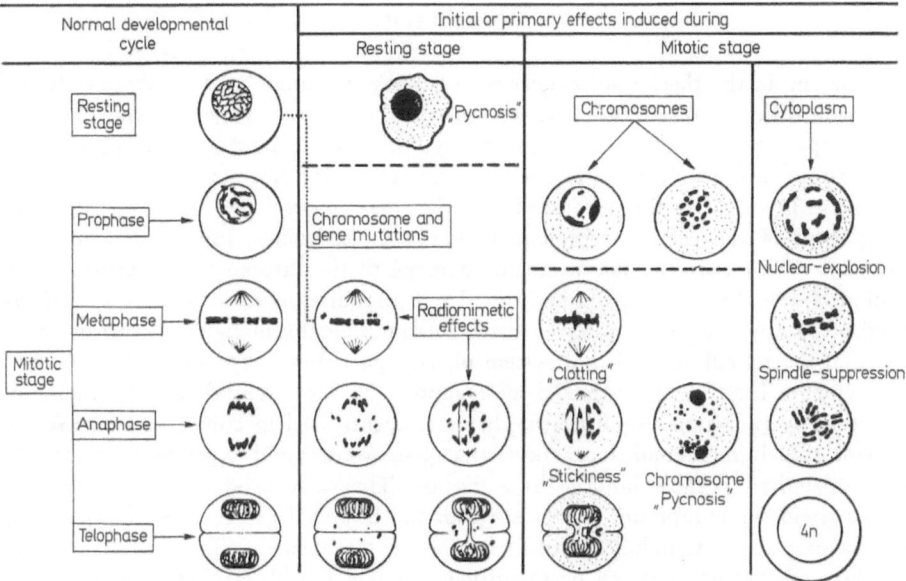

Fig. 42. Diagram showing the various chromosome injuries which can appear in dividing cells after treatment with chemical agents

preferential toxicity to dividing cells. According to the stage at which the initial damage is inflicted by these agents, the cytological injuries are of two kinds: (1) "nucleotoxic effects" — chromosome breaks and interchanges initiated in the interphase nucleus and (2) "cytotoxic effects" — physiological disturbances which are revealed in cells already in the process of mitosis by stickiness and clumping of chromosomes, and sticky anaphase bridges. These various types of cell injuries are illustrated in Fig. 42.

In the therapy of cancer it is of secondary importance whether the proliferating cells die by chromosome injuries or by cytotoxic disturbances. Under certain conditions the latter can be even more important than the true radiomimetic effects e. g. Myleran. The most serious shortcomings of alkylating agents is in their interference with DNA synthesis and their inability to distinguish between DNA synthesis of normal and malignant cells. One possibility for enhancing selectively is to make use of specific enzyme systems which are a characteristic property of particular cells and tissues, and to attack the cells through these systems. The effect of narcotics on nerve cells or of stilboestrol on the malignant prostate gland is very likely brought about by such a selective process. However, "dedifferentiation" is of common occurence in neoplastic cells, and with loss of such a characteristic constituent from the cell, the drug becomes less selective and less effective. In the search for therapeutically valuable chemical agents, the analysis of the chromosomal effects induced by the drug under test, can be a valuable method; the radiomimetic or cytotoxic injuries are visible criteria of the biochemical lesion produced by the agents, and may indicate their potential value in the therapy of cancer.

Summary

The aim in the therapy of cancer is to destroy or render inactive those cells with an uncontrolled proliferative capacity. One of the effective ways to achieve this aim is to impair beyond the point of recovery, the genetic mechanism responsible for maintaining the neoplastic behaviour of the cell, and for regulating the metabolic pathways involved in the mitotic process. Irradiation produces injury to the genetic component of the cell, as represented by the chromosomes; injury to them results in the death of the cell. The extent of damage to the chromosomes depends on the radiation dose. Beside affecting individual cells, irradiation also produces a particular kind of reaction in the connective tissue surrounding the malignant growth; in this reaction the reticulo-endothelial system plays a part. Both experimental and empirical evidence indicates that the "tissue-reaction" has an essential role in tumour destruction by radiation. Amongst the chemical agents used in clinical practice for the control of malignant conditions, alkylating agents were found to produce chromosomal injuries similar to those induced by radiation. They also produce physiological disturbances in the cytoplasmic systems, which can be lethal to the cells. By cytological studies of the events induced in cells by chemical agents, the site of primary action (nuclear or cytoplasmic) can be identified and the possible usefulness of the agents evaluated.

Conclusion

Our present day knowledge concerning the chromosomes of cancer cells may be summarized as follows: (1) in most tumours the cells have an abnormal set of chromosomes and (2) in each case the abnormality is different; no two tumours were observed with identical aneuploid chromosome patterns. There is one striking exception to the above two points: in chronic myeloid leukaemia in man, the Ph' chromosome appears to be a highly specific morphological marker for this type of malignancy, and is believed by some to participate in the causation of the disease. On the other hand, the lack of any consistency in the chromosomal anomalies observed in human tumours, and their great karyotypic variability, support the view that chromosomal changes are secondary phenomena, resulting from the neoplastic state of the cell. The mitotic abnormalities — so common in premalignant and malignant tissues, are further evidence of a disturbed intracellular metabolism, responsible for the appearance of cells in which the chromosome constitution deviates from the normal diploid state. The configuration of anomalous chromosome patterns is a decisive factor which determines whether the aneuploid cell has proliferative capacity or not. Observation shows that very drastic chromosomal anomalies are tolerated in the neoplastic tissue, because there "they matter less than elsewhere".

Studies of animal tumours, particularly those grown in the ascites form and therefore suitable for experimentation, demonstrated that cell populations of tumours are heterogeneous; they are composed of chromosome variants present in differing frequencies. The stemline cells which form the largest class amongst the chromosome variants, are considered to be responsible for the growth of the tumours, but in a changing environment they can be replaced by other cell variants. Selection experiments revealed the existence of variants in the malignant cell population which differ in many respects e. g. antigenicity, enzymatic activity as well as resistance to drugs and radiation. In some instances a relationship was established between chromosomal constitution and cellular function, in others no such correlation was found. Thus the mosaic composition of the cell population in tumours reflects genotypic differences between cells but the cell variants do not necessarily show karyotypic differences.

Chromosomal analysis of human malignant tumours provided evidence that, as in experimental animal tumours, the great majority are composed of a heterogeneous cell population. Chromosomal aneuploidy has been observed in precancerous conditions, and is considered to have a prognostic value, indicating that the lesion could progress towards a truly malignant invasive stage. In tumours correlation seems to exist between the degree and pattern of aneuploidy and the degree of malignancy; such a correlation however, occurs in a characteristic fashion for any given type of tumour. The association of particular malignancies with a constitutional chromosome anomaly, and the development of leukaemia in carriers of a familial chromosome aberration give support to the view that cells with chromosome anomalies have an enhanced susceptibility to malignant transformation. Studies of chromosome behaviour have thrown further light on the biological basis of radio- and chemotherapy. According to recent reports, chromosome analysis may be one of the methods which could be used not only to identify persons with a high risk of developing cancer, but also to detect the carcinogenic potentiality of environmental agents.

The concept that the cell populations of tumours are heterogeneous is one of the most valuable findings derived from chromosome studies. It seems that malignant growth is composed of competing clones of cells with different and continuously changing genotypes, confering the tumour with an adaptable plasticity against the environment. The bewildering karyotypic patterns reveal the multi-potentiality of the neoplastic cell; while normal cells and tissues age and die, through their inherent variability, tumour cells proliferate and survive. Chromosome studies lead to the conclusion that the law of generalization is not applicable to cancer; every cancerous growth is a specific, individual dynamic entity, whose most important characteristic lies in its cellular variability.

References

AARONSON, S. A., TODARO, G. J.: Transformation and virus growth by murine sarcoma viruses in human cells. Nature (Lond.) **225**, 458 (1970).

AL-SADI, A., BEIERWALTERS, W. H.: Sequential cytogenetic changes in the evolution of transplanted thyroid tumors to metastatic carcinoma in the Fisher rat. Cancer Res. **27**, 1831 (1967).

ARNOLD, J.: Beobachtungen über Kerntheilungen in den Zellen der Geschwülste. Virchows Arch. Abt. A Path. Anat. **78**, 279 (1879).

ATKIN, N. B.: The chromosome changes in malignancy; an assessment of their possible prognostic significance. Brit. J. Radiol. **37**, 213 (1964).

ATKIN, N. B.: Cytogenetic studies on human tumors and premalignant lesions; the emergence of aneuploid cell lines and their relationship to the process of malignant transformation in man. In "Genetic Concepts and Neoplasia". Baltimore: Williams and Wilkins Co., 1970.

ATKIN, N. B., BAKER, M. C.: Chromosome abnormalities as primary events in human malignant disease; evidence from marker chromosomes. J. nat. Cancer Inst. **36**, 539 (1966).

AUERSPERG, N., COREY, M. J., WORTH, A.: Chromosomes of preinvasive lesions of the human uterine cervix. Cancer Res. **27**, 1394 (1967).

BARSKI, G., SORIEUL, S., CORNEFERT, F.: Production dans des (sic) cultures *in vitro* deux souches cellulaires en association, de cellules de caractère "Hybride". C. R. Acad. Sci. (Paris) **251**, 1825 (1960).

BAUKE, J.: Examples of clonal evolution in chronic myeloid leukaemia. Exc. med.; Int. Cong. Series no. **233**, 23 (1971).

BAYREUTHER, K.: Der Chromosomenbestand des Ehrlich-Ascites-Tumors der Maus. Z. f. Naturforschung **7**, 554 (1952).

BAYREUTHER, K.: Chromosomes in the primary neoplastic growth. Nature (Lond.) **186**, 6 (1960 a).

BAYREUTHER, K.: Chromosome behaviour in tumors; Discussion. In "Cell Physiol. of Neoplasia" Univ. Texas, Austin: 1960 b.

BENEDICT, W. F., PORTER, J. H., BROWN, C. D., DOYLE, G. J.: Chromosomes in malignancy. Lancet I, 922 (1968).

BERGER, R. Chromosomes et leucémies humaines. La notion d'evolution clonale. Ann. Génét. **8**, 70 (1965).

BIESELE, J. J., BIEDLER, J. L., HUTCHINSON, D.: The chromosomal status of drug resistant sublines of mouse leukaemia. In "Genetics and Cancer". Univ. Texas, Houston. 1961.

BITTNER, J. J.: Some possible effects of nursing on the mammary gland tumor incidence in mice. Science **84**, 162 (1936).

BLAKESLEE, A. F.: Variation in *Datura* due to changes in chromosome number. Amer. Nat. **56**, 16 (1922).

BODDINGTON, M. M., SPRIGGS, A. I., WOLFENDALE, M. R.: Cytogenetic abnormalities in carcinoma *in-situ* and dysplasias of the uterine cervix. Brit. med. J. I, 154 (1965).

BOTTOMLEY, R. H., TRAINER, A. L., GRIFFIN, M. J.: Enzymatic and chromosomal characterization of HeLa variants. J. Cell Biol. **41**, 306 (1969).

BOVERI, T.: Beitrag zum Studium des Chromatin in den Epithelzellen der Carcinome. Beitr. Path. Anat. **14**, 249 (1912).

BOVERI, T.: Zur Frage der Entstehung maligner Tumoren. Jena: Gustav Fischer 1914.

Boyd, J. T., Court-Brown, W. M., Vennart, J., Woodcock, G. E.: Chromosome studies on women formerly employed as luminous-dial painters. Brit. med. J. I, 377 (1966).

Bridges, C. B.: Non-disjunction as proof of the chromosome theory of heredity. Genetics 1, 107 (1916).

Brookes, P., Lawley, P. D.: Evidence for the action of alkylating agents on deoxyribonucleic acid. Exp. Cell Res. Suppl. 9, 521 (1963).

Bruyn De, W. M., Hansen-Melander, E.: The chromosomes of the M. B. Lymphosarcoma. Hereditas (Lund) 44, 558 (1958).

Carr, D. H.: Chromosome studies in abortuses and stillborn infants. Lancet II, 603 (1963).

Caspersson, T., Zech, L., Johansson, C., Modest, E.J.: Identification of human chromosomes by DNA-binding fluorescent agents. Chromosoma (Berl.) 30, 215 (1970).

Castoldi, G., Yam, L. T., Mitus, W. J., Crosby, W. H.: Chromosomal studies in erythro-leukaemia and chronic erythremic myelosis. Blood 31, 202 (1968).

Cellier, K. M., Kirkland, J. A., Stanley, M. A.: Statistical analysis of cytogenetic data in cervical neoplasia. J. nat. Cancer Inst. 44, 1221 (1970).

Chernay, P. R., Hsu, L. Y. F., Streicher, H., Hirschhorn, K.: Human chromosome identification by differential staining: G-group (21—22—Y). Cytogenet. 10, 219 (1971).

Chu, E. H. Y., Giles, N. H.: Comparative chromosomal studies on mammalian cells in culture I. The HeLa strain and its mutant clonal derivatives. J. nat. Cancer Inst. 20, 383 (1958).

Ciuffo, G.: Innesto positivo con filtrate di verruca vulgare. G. ital. Mal. vener. 42, 12 (1907).

Cox, D., Yuncken, C., Spriggs, A. J.: Minute chromatin bodies in malignant tumours of childhood. Lancet II, 55 (1965).

Crick, F.: General model for the chromosomes of higher organisms. Nature (Lond.) 243, 25 (1971).

Diehl, V., Henle, G., Henle, W., Kohn, G.: Demonstration of a Herpes group virus in cultures of peripheral leukocytes from patients with infectious mononucleosis. J. Virology 2, 663 (1968).

Earle, W. R.: Production of malignancy in vitro IV. The mouse fibroblast cultures and changes seen in the living cells. J. nat. Cancer Inst. 4, 165 (1943).

Eddy, B. E., Borman, G. S., Berkeley, W. H., Young, R. D.: Tumors induced in hamsters by injection of Rhesus monkey kidney cell extracts. Proc. Soc. exp. Biol. (N. Y.) 107, 191 (1961).

Ellerman, V., Bang, O.: Experimentelle Leukämie bei Hühnern. Zbl. Bakt., I, Abt. Ref. 46, 595 (1908).

Engel, E., McGee, B. J., Hartmann, R. C., Engel de Montmollin, M.: Two leukaemic peripheral blood stemlines during acute transformation of chronic myelogenous leukaemias in a D/D translocation carrier. Cytogenet. 4, 157 (1965).

Enterline, H. T., Arvan, D. A.: Chromosome constitution of adenoma and adenocarcinoma of the colon. Cancer (N. Y.) 20, 1746 (1967).

Epstein, M. A., Achong, B. G., Barr, Y. M.: Virus particles in cultured lymphoblasts from Burkitt's lymphoma. Lancet I, 702 (1964).

Farmer, J. B., Moore, J. E. S., Walker, C. E.: On resemblance exhibited between cells of malignant growth in man and those of normal reproductive tissue. Proc. roy. Soc. B. 72, 499 (1903).

Ferrier, P. E., Ferrier, S. A., Scharer, K. O., Genton, N. Hedinger, C., Klein, D. J.: Disturbed gonadal differentiation in a child with XO/XY/XYY mosaicism; relationship with gonadoblastoma. Helv. paediat. Acta 22, (5) 479 (1967).

Fitzgerald, P. H., Hamer, J. W.: Third case of chronic lymphocytic leukaemia in a carrier of the inherited Ch' chromosome. Brit. med. J. III, 752 (1969).

Fjelde, A., Levan, A., Rask-Nielsen, R.: The chromosomes of four transplantable murine plasma cell leukaemias characterized by varying pathological serum protein changes and/or amyloid formation. Hereditas (Lund) 48, 630 (1962).

Ford, C. E., Hamerton, J. L., Mole, R. H.: Chromosomal changes in the primary and transplanted reticular neoplasms of the mouse. J. cell. comp. Physiol. 52, 235 (1958).

Ford, C. E.: Jones, K. W., Miller, O. J., Mittwoch, V., Penrose, L. S., Ridler, M., Shapiro, A.: Chromosomes in a patient showing both mongolism and the Klinefelter syndrome. Lancet I, 709 (1959).

FORD, C. E., CLARKE, C. M.: Cytogenetic evidence of clonal proliferation in primary reticular neoplasms. Canad. Cancer Conf. 5, 129 (1963).

FORNI, A., MOREO, L.: Cytogenetic studies in a case of benzene leukaemia. Europ. J. Cancer 3, 251 (1967).

FRACCARO, M., KAIJSER, K., LINDSTEN, J.: Chromosomal abnormalities in father and mongol child. Lancet I, 724 (1960).

FRACCARO, M., MANNINI, A., TIEPOLO, L., GERLI, M., ZARA, C.: Karyotypic clonal evolution in a cystic adenoma of the ovary. Lancet I, 613 (1968).

FRAUMENI, J. F., Jr., MILLER, R. W.: Epidemiology of human leukaemia; recent observations. J. nat. Cancer Inst. 38, 593 (1967).

GALLO, R. C., STRINGER, S. J., TING, R. C.: RNA dependent DNA polymerase of human acute leukaemic cells. Nature (Lond.) 228, 927 (1970).

GEY, G. O., COFFMAN, W. D., KUBICEK, M. T.: Tissue culture studies of the proliferative capacity of cervical carcinoma and normal epithelium. Cancer Res. 12, 264 (1952).

GILBERT, G. W., MULDAL, S.: Measurement and computer system for karyotyping human and other cells. Nature (New Biol.) 230, 203 (1971).

GLÄSS, E.: Die Chromosomenzahlen in der durch Buttergelbverfütterung krebsig entarteten Rattenleber. Z. Krebsforsch. 63, 362 (1960).

GOFMAN, J. W., MINKLER, J. L., TANDY, R. K.: "A specific common chromosomal pathway for the origin of human malignancy". US Dept. of Commerce, Springfield, Virginia, USA (1967).

GOH, K.: Large acrocentric chromosomes associated with human malignancies; Possible mechanism of establishing clones of cells. Arch. Internat. Med. 122, 241 (1968).

GOH, K., SWISHER, S. N.: Identical twins and chronic myelocytic leukaemia. Arch. Internat. Med. 115, 475 (1965).

GRAY, L. H., CONGER, A. D., EBERT, M., HORNSBY, S., SCOTT, O. C.: Concentration of oxygen dissolved in tissues at a time of irradiation as a factor in radiotherapy. Brit. J. Radiol. 26, 638 (1953).

GROSS, L.: "Spontaneous" leukaemia developing in C3H mice following inoculation in infancy, with AK-leukaemic extracts, or AK-embryos. Proc. Soc. exp. Biol. (N. Y.) 76, 27 (1951).

GROUCHY DE, J., DE NAVA, C., CANTU, J.-M., BILSKI-PASQUIER, G., BOUSSER, J.: Models for clonal evolutions: A study of chronic myelogeneous leukaemia. Amer. J. hum. Genet. 18, 485 (1966).

GROUCHY DE, J., DE NAVA, C., FEINGOLD, J., BILSKI-PASQUIER, G., BOUSSER, J.: Onze observations d'un modèle précis d'evolution caryotypique au cours de la leucémie myéloide chronique. Europ. J. Cancer 4, 481 (1968).

GUNZ, F. W., FITZGERALD, P. H., ADAMS, A.: An abnormal chromosome in chronic lymphocytic leukaemia. Brit. med. J. II, 1097 (1962).

HADDOW, A., TIMMIS, E. G. M.: Myleran in chronic myeloid leukaemia I. Chemical constitution and biological action. Lancet I, 207 (1953).

HAKALA, M. T., ISHIHARA, T.: Chromosomal constitution and amethopterin resistance in cultured mouse cells. Cancer Res. 22, part I, 987 (1962).

HALDANE, J. B. S.: Genetical evidence for cytological abnormality in man. J. Genet. 26, 341 (1932).

HAMMUDA, P., QUAGLINO, D., HAYHOE, F. G. J.: Blastic crisis in chronic granulocytic leukaemia — Cytochemical, cytogenetic and autoradiographic studies in four cases. Brit. med. J. I, 1275 (1964).

HANSEMANN VON, D.: Über Asymmetrische Zelltheilung in Epithelkrebsen und deren biologische Bedeutung. Virchow's Arch. path. Anat. 119, 299 (1890).

HANSEN-MELANDER, E., KULLANDER, S., MELANDER, Y.: Chromosome analysis of a human ovarian cystocarcinoma in the ascites form. J. nat. Cancer Inst. 16, 1067 (1956).

HARNDEN, D. G., LANGLANDS, A. O., McBEATH, S., O'RIORDAN, M.: FAED, M. J. W.: The frequency of constitutional chromosome abnormalities in patients with malignant disease. Europ. J. Cancer 5, 605 (1969).

HAUSCHKA, T. S.: Correlation of chromosomal and physiologic changes in tumors. J. cell. comp. Physiol. 52, suppl. 1, 197 (1958).

HAUSCHKA, T. S.: The chromosome in ontogeny and oncogeny. Cancer Res. 21, 957 (1961).

HAUSCHKA, T. S., Levan, A.: Inverse relationship between chromosome ploidy and host specificity in sixteen transplantable tumors. Exp. Cell Res. 4, 457 (1953).

HAUSCHKA, T. S., LEVAN, A.: Cytologic and functional characterization of single cell clones isolated from Krebs — 2 and Ehrlich Ascites tumors. J. nat. Cancer Inst. 21, 77 (1958).

HAUSCHKA, T. S., WEISS, L., HOLDBRIDGE, B. A., CUDNEY, T. L., ZUMPFT, M., PLANINSEK, J. A.: Karyotypic and surface features of murine TA3 carcinoma cells during immunoselection in mice and rats. J. nat. Cancer Inst. 47, 343 (1971).

HELLSTRÖM, K. E.: Chromosomal studies on primary methylcholanthrene-induced sarcomas in the mouse. J. nat. Cancer Inst. 23, 1019 (1959).

HELLSTRÖM, K. E.: Chromosomal studies on diethylstilboestrol-induced testicular tumors in mice. J. nat. Cancer Inst. 26, 707 (1961).

HELLSTRÖM, K. E., HELLSTRÖM, I., SJÖGREN, H. O.: Further studies on karyotypes of a variety of primary and transplanted mouse polyoma tumours. J. nat. Cancer Inst. 31, 1239 (1963).

HITOTSUMACHI, S., RABINOWITZ, Z., SACHS, L.: Chromosomal control of reversion in transformed cells. Nature (Lond.) 231, 511 (1971).

HOUSTON, E. W., RITZMANN, S. E., LEVIN, W. C.: Chromosomal aberrations common to three types of monoclonal gammopathies. Blood 29, 214 (1967).

HSU, T. C.: Cytological studies of HeLa I. Observations of mitosis and chromosomes. Tex. Rep. Biol. Med. 12, 833 (1954 a).

HSU, T. C.: Mammalian chromosomes in vitro; IV. Some human neoplasms. J. nat. Cancer Inst. 14, 905 (1954 b).

HSU, T. C.: Mammalian chromosomes in vitro; XI. Variability among progenies of a single cell. Univ. Texas Publ. 5914; 129 (1959).

HSU, T. C.: Mammalian chromosomes in vitro; XIII. Cyclic and directional changes of population structure. J. nat. Cancer Inst. 25, 1339 (1960).

HSU, T. C.: Chromosomal evolution in cell populations. Int. Rev. Cytol. 12, 69 (1961).

HSU, T. C., MOORHEAD, P. S.. Mammalian chromosomes in vitro; VII. Heteroploidy in human cell strains. J. nat. Cancer Inst. 18, 463 (1957).

HSU, T. C., KELLOG, D. S.: Genetics of in vitro cells. In "Genetics and Cancer". Univ. Texas Austin: (1959).

HUANG, C. C., MINOWADA, J., SMITH, R. T., OSUNKOYA, B. O.: Revaluation of relationship between C chromosome marker and Epstein-Barr virus: chromosome and immunofluorescence analyses of 16 human hematopoietic cell lines. J. nat. Cancer Inst. 45, 815 (1970).

HUEBNER, R. J., TODARO, G. J.: Oncogenes of RNA tumor viruses as determinants of cancer. Proc. nat. Acad. Sci. (Wash.) 64, 1087 (1969).

HUGHES, D. T.: The role of chromosomes in the characterization of human neoplasms. Europ. J. Cancer 1, 233 (1965).

ISHIBASHI, K.: Studies on the number of cells necessary for the transplantation of Yoshida sarcoma. Gann, 41, 1 (1950).

ISHIHARA, T., MOORE, G. E., SANDBERG, A. A.: Chromosome constitution of cells in effusions of cancer patients. J. nat. Cancer Inst. 27, 893 (1961).

ISHIHARA, T.: The in vitro chromosome constitution of cells from human tumors. Cancer Res. 22, 375 (1962).

ISHIHARA, T., SANDBERG, A. A.: Chromosome constitution of diploid and pseudo-diploid cells in effusions of cancer patients. Cancer (N. Y.) 16, 885 (1963).

JOLLES, B., KOLLER, P. C.: The role of connective tissue in the radiation reaction of tumours. Brit. J. Cancer 4, 298 (1950).

JOLLES, B., KOLLER, P. C.: Radiation in tumours with fractionation in space. Acta Un. int. contra Canc. 9, 51 (1953).

JONES, H. W., DAVIS, H. J., FROST, J. K., PARK, In-Jo, SALIMI, R., TSENG, P-Y., WOODRUFF, J. D.: The value of the assay of chromosomes in the diagnosis of cervical neoplasia. Amer. J. Obstet. Gynec. 102, 624 (1968).

KATO, R.: The chromosomes of forty-two primary Rous sarcomas of the Chinese hamster. Hereditas (Lund) 59 (I), 63 (1968).

KAY, H. E. M., LAWLER, S. D., MILLARD, R. E.: The chromosomes of polycythaemia vera. Brit. J. Haemat. 12, 507 (1966).

KEMP, N. H., STAFFORD, J. L., TANNER, R.: Aetiology of leukaemias. Lancet I, 152 (1963).

KIOSSOGLOU, K. A., MITUS, W. J., DAMASHEK, W.: Chromosomal aberrations in acute leukaemia. Blood 26, 610 (1965).

KLEBS, E.: Allgemeine Pathologie. Jena (1889).

KLEIN, G., KLEIN, E.: Cytogenetics of experimental tumors. In "Genetics and Cancer". Univ. Texas, Houston (1961).

KOHN, G., MELLMAN, W. J., MOORHEAD, P. S., LOFTUS, J., HENLE, G.: Involvement of C-group chromosomes in five Burkitt lymphoma cell lines. J. nat. Cancer Inst. 38, 209 (1967).

KOLLER, P. C.: The genetical and mechanical properties of sex chromosomes III. Man. Proc. roy. Soc. Edinb. B 2, 194 (1937).

KOLLER, P. C.: Asynapsis in *Pisum sativum*. J. Genet. 36, 275 (1938).

KOLLER, P. C.: Origin of malignant tumour cells. Nature (Lond.) 151, 244 (1943).

KOLLER, P. C.: A new technique for mitosis in tumours. Nature (Lond.) 149, 193 (1942).

KOLLER, P. C.: Abnormal mitosis in tumours. Brit. J. Cancer 1, 38 (1947 a).

KOLLER, P. C.: Experimental modification of the nucleic acid systems in the cell. Symp. Soc. exp. Biol. Symposia I. Nucleic Acids. 270 (1947 b).

KOLLER, P. C.: Dicentric chromosomes in a rat tumour induced by an aromatic nitrogen mustard. Heredity 6, suppl. 181 (1953).

KOLLER, P. C.: Biological Basis of Radiotherapy. In Cancer 5, Ed.: R. W. Raven, Butterworth, London (1959).

KOLLER, P. C.: Chromosome behaviour in tumors; Readjustments to Boveri's theory. In Cell Physiol. of Neoplasia, Univ. Texas Austin (1960).

KOLLER, P. C., SMITHERS, D. W.: Cytological analysis of the response of malignant tumours to irradiation as an approach to a biological basis for dosage in radiotherapy. Brit. J. Radiol. 19, 89 (1946).

KOLLER, P. C., WAYMOUTH, C.: Observations on intracellular leucocytes in tissue cultures of a rat tumour. J. roy. micr. Soc. 72, 173 (1952).

KÖNIGSBERG, A., NITOWSKY, H.: Studies of the karyotype of clonal strains of Chang liver in alkaline-phosphatase activity. J. nat. Cancer Inst. 29, 699 (1962).

KROLL, W., SCHLESINGER, K.: Chromosome studies in an infant with acute erythremic myelosis. Blood 35, 282 (1970).

KROMPECHER, E.: Über Zellteilung. Zbl. allg. Path. path Anat. 13, 273 (1902).

LA COUR, L.: Improvements in everyday technique in plant cytology. J. roy. micr. Soc. 51, 119 (1931).

LAMB, D.: Correlation of chromosome counts with histological appearances and prognosis in transitional cell carcinoma of the bladder. Brit. med. J. I, 273 (1967).

LAWLER, S. D., PENTYCROSS, C. R., REEVES, B. R.: Chromosomes and transformation of lymphocytes in lymphoproliferative disorders. Brit. med. J. IV, 213 (1968).

LEJEUNE, J., TURPIN, R., GAUTIER, M.: La mongolisme, premier example d'aberration autosomique humaine. Ann. Génét. 1, 41 (1959).

LEJEUNE, J., BERGER, R., HAINES, M., LAFOURCARDE, J., VIALATTE, J., SATGE, P., TURPIN, R.: Constitution d'un clone a 54 chromosomes au cours d'une leucoblastose congenitale chez une enfant mongolienne. C. R. Acad. Sci. (Paris). 256, 1195 (1963).

LEJEUNE, J., BERGER, R., CAILLE, B., TURPIN, R.: Evolution d'une leucémie myeloide chronique. Ann. Génét. 8, 44 (1965).

LETTRE, H.: Einige Beobachtungen über das Wachstum des Mäuse-Ascites Tumors und seine Beeinflussung. Z. Physiol. Chem. 268, 59 (1941).

LEVAN, A.: Significance of polyploidy for the evolution of mouse tumors. Exp. Cell Res. 11, 613 (1956 a).

LEVAN, A.: Chromosome studies on some human tumors and tissues of normal origin, grown *in vivo* and *in vitro* at the Sloan Kettering Institute. Cancer (N. Y.) 9, 648 (1956 b).

LEVAN, A., HAUSCHKA, T. S.: Chromosome numbers of three mouse ascites tumors. Hereditas (Lund) 38, 251 (1952).

LEVAN, A., HAUSCHKA, T. S.: Endomitotic reduplication mechanism in ascites tumors of the mouse. J. nat. Cancer Inst. 14, 1 (1953).

LEVAN, A., BIESELE, J. J.: Role of chromosomes in cancerogenesis as studied in serial tissue culture of mammalian cells. Ann. N. Y. Acad. Sci 71, 1022 (1958).

LITTBRAND, B., RÉVÉSZ, L.: The effect of oxygen on cellular survival and recovery after radiation. Brit. J. Radiol. **42**, 914 (1969).

LOEWENTHAL, H., JAHN, G.: Übertragungsversuche mit carcinomatöser Mäuse Ascites-Flüssigkeit und ihr Verhalten gegen physikalische und chemische Einwirkungen. Z. Krebsforsch. **37**, 439 (1932).

LUBS, A., KOTLER, S.: The prognostic significance of chromosome abnormalities in colon tumours. Ann. intern. Med. **67**, 328 (1967).

MACEK, M., SEIDEL, E. H., LEWIS, R. T., BRUNSCHWIG, J. P.: Cytogenetic studies of EB-virus-positive and EB-virus-negative lymphoblastoid cell lines. Cancer Res. **31**, 308 (1971).

MAKINO, S.: Further evidence favoring the concept of the stem cell in ascites tumors of rats. Ann. N. Y. Acad. Sci. **14**, 818 (1956).

MAKINO, S., KANO, K.: Cytological studies of tumors XIV. Isolation of single-cell clones from a mixed-cell tumor of the rat. J. nat. Cancer Inst. **15**, 1165 (1955).

MAKINO, S., ISHIHARA, T., TONOMURA, A.: Cytological studies of tumors; XXVII. The chromosomes of thirty human tumors. Z. Krebsforsch. **63**, 184 (1959).

MAKINO, S., SASAKI, M. S., TONOMURA, A.: Cytological studies of tumors XL. Chromosome studies in fifty-two human tumors. J. nat. Cancer Inst. **32**, 741 (1964).

MARIN, G., LITTLEFIELD, J. W.: Selection of morphologically normal cell lines from Polyoma-transformed BHK21/13 hamster fibroblasts. J. Virol. **2**, 69 (1968).

MARK, J.: Chromosome analysis of ninety-one primary Rous sarcomas in the mouse. Hereditas (Lund) **57**, 23 (1967).

MARTINEAU, M.: A similar marker chromosome in testicular tumours. Lancet I, 836 (1966).

McDOUGALL, J. K.: Effects of adenoviruses on the chromosomes of normal human cells and cells trisomic for an E chromosome. Nature (Lond.) **225**, 456 (1970).

McMICHAEL, H., WAGNER, J. E., NOWELL, P. C., HUNGERFORD, D.: Chromosome studies of virus-induced rabbit papillomas and derived primary carcinomas. J. nat. Cancer Inst. **31** (5), 1197 (1963).

MERZ, T., EL-MAHDI, A. M., PREMPREE, T.: Unusual chromosomes and malignant disease. Lancet I, 337 (1968).

MILES, C. P.: Chromosome analysis of solid tumors. I. twenty-eight non-epithelial tumors. Cancer (N. Y.) **20**, 1253 (1967).

MILES, C. P.: Chromosome analysis of solid tumors. II. twenty-six epithelial tumors. Cancer (N. Y.) **20**, 1274 (1967).

MILLER, R. W., TODARO, G. J.: Viral transformation of cells from persons with high risk of cancer. Lancet I, 81 (1969).

MOORHEAD, P. S.: Virus effects on host chromosomes. In "Genetic Concepts and Neoplasia". Williams and Wilkins Co. Baltimore: (1970).

MORIWAKI, K., IMAI, H. T., YOSIDA, T. H.: Polyploidization and protein synthesis in mammalian cells. Jap. J. Genetics **44**, suppl. 1, 71 (1969).

MUKERJEE, D., TRUJILLO, J. M., CORK, A., BOWEN, J. M.: Genetic susceptibility of human cells to transformation by oncogenic viruses. Excerpt. Med. Int. Cong. Serial no. **233**, 128 (1971).

MULDAL, S., ELEJALDE, R., HARVEY, P. W.: Specific chromosome anomaly associated with autonomous and cancerous development in man. Nature (Lond.) **229**, 48 (1971).

NOWELL, P. C.: Prognostic value of marrow chromosome studies in human "Preleukaemia". Arch. Path. **80**, 205 (1965).

NOWELL, P. C.: Marrow chromosome studies in "Preleukaemia". Further correlation with clinical course. Cancer (N. Y.) **28**, 513 (1971).

NOWELL, P. C., HUNGERFORD, D. A.: A minute chromosome in human chronic granulocytic leukaemia. Science **132**, 1197 (1960).

NOWELL, P. C., HUNGERFORD, D. A.: Chromosome changes in human leukaemia and a tentative assessment of their significance. Ann. N. Y. Acad. Sci. **113**, 654 (1964).

NOWELL, P. C., MORRIS, H. P., POTTER, V. R.: Chromosomes of "minimal deviation" hepatomas and some other transplantable rat tumors. Cancer Res. **27**, 1565 (1967).

OHNO, S., KOVACS, E. T., KINOSITA, R.: On the X-chromosomes of the mouse mammary carcinoma cells. Exp. Cell Res. **16**, 462 (1959).

O'RIORDAN, M. L., ROBINSON, J. A., BUCKTON, K. E., EVANS, H. J.: Distinguishing between the chromosomes involved in Down's syndrome (Trisomy-21) and chronic myeloid leukaemia (Ph') by fluorescence. Nature (Lond.) 230, 167 (1971).

PATAU, K.: Chromosomal abnormalities in Waldenström's macroglobulinaemia. Lancet II, 600 (1961).

PAYNE, F. E., SCHMICKEL, R. D.: Susceptibility of trisomic and of triploid human fibroblasts to Simian Virus 40 (SV40). Nature (New Biol.) 230, 190 (1971).

PEDERSEN, B.: Ph'-disomy and prognosis in chronic myelogeneous leukaemia. Acta haemat. (Basel) 39, 102 (1968).

PEDERSEN, B.: Karyotype evolution in human leukaemia — relation between karyotypes cellular phenotypes and clinical progression. Exc. Med. Int. Cong. Series no. 233, 8 (1971).

PENROSE, L. S.: Maternal age, order of birth and developmental abnormalities. Ann. Eugen. (Lond.) 13, 25 (1939).

PETTERSEN, G., BONNIER, G.: Inherited sex mosaic in man. Hereditas (Lund) 23, 49 (1937).

POLANI, P. E., BRIGGS, J. H., FORD, C. E., CLARKE, C. M., BERG, J. M.: A mongol girl with 46 chromosomes. Lancet I, 721 (1960).

POLLACK, R., WOLMAN, S., VOGEL, A.: Reversion of virus-transformed cell lines: Hyperploidy accompanies retention of viral genes. Nature (Lond.) 228, 938 (1970).

POPP, S., LIZZI, F.: Philadelphia chromosome in acute lymphocytic leukaemia. Blood 36, 353 (1970).

PORTER, J. H., BENEDICT, W. F., BROWN, C. D., PAUL, B.: Recent advances in molecular pathology; A review. Some aspects of chromosome changes in cancer. Exp. and Molec. Pathol. 11, 340 (1969).

POTTER VAN, R.: Biochemical studies on minimal deviation hepatomas. In "Cellular Control Mechanism and Cancer". Eds.: P. Emmelot and O. Muhlbock. Elsevier Pub. Co. Amsterdam-London-New York (1964).

PRIGOGINA, E. L., STAVROVSKAJA, A. A., KAKPAKOVA, E. S., STRELJUCHINA, N. V., ZAKHAROV, A. F., LELIKOVA, G. P., CHUDINA, A. P., POGOSIANZ, E. E.: Congenital chromosome abnormalities and leukaemia. Lancet II, 524 (1970).

RABINOWITZ, Z., SACHS, L.: Control of the reversion of properties in transformed cells. Nature (Lond.) 225, 136 (1970).

RAPP, F., BUTEL, J. S.: The virus genome and transformation of mammalian cells. In "Genetic Concepts and Neoplasia". Williams and Wilkins Co., Baltimore (1970).

RÉVÉSZ, L., GLAS, U., HILDING, G.: Relationship between chromosome number and radiosensitivity of tumour cells. Nature (Lond.) 198, 260 (1963).

RHYNAS, P. O. W., NEWCOMBE, H. B.: A heritable change in radiation resistance of strain L mouse cells. Radiat. Res. 21, 326 (1961).

RICH, M. A., TSUCHIDA, R., SIEGLER, R.: Chromosome aberrations: their role in the etiology of murine leukemia. Science 146, 252 (1964).

RICHART, R. M., CORFMAN, P. A.: Chromosome number and morphology of a human preinvasive neoplasm. Science 144, 65 (1964).

RICHART, R. M., WILBANKS, G. D.: The chromosomes of human intraepithelial neoplasia: Report of 14 cases of cervical intraepithelial neoplasia and review. Cancer Res. 26, 60 (1966).

RIGBY, C. C.: Chromosome studies in ten testicular tumours. Brit. J. Cancer 22, 480 (1968).

ROUS, P.: A transmissible avian neoplasm. J. exp. Med. 12, 696 (1910).

ROWLEY, J. D., BODMER, W. F.: Relationship of centromeric heterochromatin to fluorescent banding patterns of metaphase chromosomes in the mouse. Nature (Lond.) 231, 503 (1971).

RUDKIN, G., HUNGERFORD, D. A., NOWELL, P.: DNA contents of chromosome Ph' and chromosome 21 in human chronic granulocytic leukaemia. Science 144, 1229 (1964).

SANDBERG, A. A.: The chromosomes and causation of human cancer and leukaemia. Cancer Res. 26, 2064 (1966).

SANDBERG, A. A., ISHIHARA, T., MOORE, G. E., PICKREN, J. W.: Unusually high polyploidy in a human cancer. Cancer 16, 1246 (1963).

SANDBERG, A. A., YAMADA, K., KIKUCHI, Y., TAKAGI, N.: Chromosomes and causation of human cancer and leukaemia III. Karyotypes of cancerous effusions. Cancer (N. Y.) 20, 1099 (1967).

SANDBERG, A. A., TAKAGI, N., SOFUNI, T.: Chromosomes and causation of human cancer and leukaemia. V. Karyotypic aspects of acute leukaemia. Cancer (N. Y.) **22**, 1268 (1968 a).

SANDBERG, A. A., BROSS, J. D. J., TAKAGI, N., SCHMIDT, M. L.: Chromosomes and causation of human cancer IV. Vectorial analysis. Cancer (N. Y.) **21**, 77 (1968 b).

SANDBERG, A. A., HOSSFELD, D. K.: Chromosomal abnormalities in human neoplasia. Ann. Rev. Med. **21**, 379 (1970).

SAWITSKY, A., BLOOM, D., GERMAN, J.: Chromosome breakage in acute leukaemia in congenital telengiectatic erythema and stunted growth. Ann. intern. Med. **65**, 487 (1966).

SCHNEIDER, G., STRECHER, G., OBRECHT, P., MERKER, H.: Atypical Ph' chromosome by pericentric inversion. Lancet **II**, 1367 (1967).

SCOLNICK, E. M., AARONSON, S. A., TODARO, G. J., PARK, W. P.: RNA-dependent DNA polymerase activity in mammalian cells. Nature (Lond.) **229**, 318 (1971).

SHOPE, R. E.: A filterable virus causing tumor-like condition in rabbits and its relationship to virus myxomatosum. J. exp. Med. **56**, 803 (1932).

SPIERS, A. S. D., BAIKIE, A. G.: Cytogenetic studies in the malignant lymphomas and related neoplasms. Cancer (N. Y.) **22**, 193 (1968 a).

SPIERS, A. S. D., BAIKIE, A. G.: Cytogenetic evolution and clonal proliferation in acute transformation and chronic granulocytic leukaemia. Brit. J. Cancer **22**, 192 (1968 b).

SPRIGGS, A. I., BODDINGTON, M. M., CLARKE, C. M.: Carcinoma *in-situ* of the cervix uteri: some cytogenetic observations. Lancet **I**, 1383 (1962).

STEELE, C. M.: Non-identity of apparently similar chromosome aberrations in human lymphoblastoid cell lines. Nature (Lond.) **33**, 555 (1971).

STEENIS VAN, H.: Chromosomes and cancer. Nature (Lond.) **209**, 819 (1966).

STEWART, A., WEBB, J., HEWITT, D.: A survey of childhood malignancies. Brit. med. J. **I**, 1495 (1958).

STEWART, S. E., EDDY, B. E., BORGESE, N.: Neoplasms in mice inoculated with a tumor agent carried in tissue culture. J. nat. Cancer Inst. **20**, 1223 (1958).

STICH, H. F.: Mosaic composition of preneoplastic lesions and malignant neoplasms. Exp. Cell Res. **9**, 277 (1963).

STICH, H. F., WAKONIG, R., AXELRAD, A. A.: Chromosome complement of spontaneous leukaemia in AKR mice. Nature (Lond.) **184**, suppl. 13, 998 (1959).

SWIFT, M. R., HIRSCHHORN, K.: Fanconi's anaemia inherited susceptibility to chromosome breakage in various tissues. Ann. intern. Med. **65**, 496 (1966).

TEMIN, H. M., MIZUTANI, S.: RNA-dependent DNA-polymerase in virions of Rous sarcoma virus. Nature (Lond.) **226**, 1211 (1970).

THOMLINSON, R. H.: Modern trends in Radiotherapy. Eds.: T. J. Dceley and C. A. P. Wood. Butterworth, London (1967).

TJIO, J. H., LEVAN, A.: A comparative idiogram analysis of the rat and Yoshida ascites sarcoma. Hereditas (Lund) **42**, 218 (1956).

TJIO, J. H., ÖSTERGREN, G.: The chromosomes of primary mammary carcinomas in milk virus strains of the mouse. Hereditas (Lund) **44**, 451 (1958).

TODARO, G. J., GREEN, H., SWIFT, M. R.: Human diploid fibroblasts transformed with SV-40 or hybrid Adeno-7 x SV-40. Science **153**, 1252 (1966).

TODARO, G. J., MARTIN, G. M.: Increased susceptibility of Down's syndrome fibroblasts to transformation by SV-40. Proc. Soc. exp. Biol. Med. **124**, 1232 (1967).

TOEWS, H. A., KATAYAMA, K. P., MASUKAWA, T., LEWISON, E. F.: Chromosomes of benign and malignant lesions of the breast. Cancer (N. Y.) **22**, 1296 (1968).

TRENTIN, J. J., YABE, Y., TAYLOR, G.: The quest for human cancer viruses. Science **137**, 835 (1962).

TUDWAY, R. C.: Precision and the imponderables in cancer treatment. Brit. J. Radiol. **44**, 821 (1971).

WAKONIG-VAARTAJA, R.: A human tumour with identifiable cells as evidence for the mutation theory. Brit. J. Cancer **16**, 616 (1962).

WAKONIG-VAARTAJA, R., KIRKLAND, J. A.: A correlated chromosomal and histopathological study of preinvasive lesions of the cervix. Cancer (N. Y.) **18**, 1101 (1965).

WAKONIG-VAARTAJA, R., HUGHES, D. T.: Chromosomal anomalies in dysplasia, carcinoma *in situ* and carcinoma of the cervix uteri. Lancet **II**, 756 (1965).

WAKONIG-VAARTAJA, R., HUGHES, D. T.: Chromosome studies in 36 gynaecological tumours: of the cervix, corpus uteri, ovary, vagina and vulva. Europ. J. Cancer **3**, 263 (1967).

WATSON, J. D., CRICK, F. H. C.: Molecular structure of nucleic acids: a structure for deoxyribose nucleic acid. Nature (Lond.) **171**, 737 (1953).

WEISS, M.: Further studies on loss of T-antigen from somatic hybrids between mouse cells and SV40-transformed human cells. Proc. nat. Acad. Sci. (Wash.) **66**, 79 (1970).

WEISS, M., GREEN, H.: Human-mouse hybrid cell lines containing partial elements of human chromosomes and functioning human genes. Proc. nat. Acad. Sci. (Wash.) **58**, 1104 (1967).

WHANG-PENG, J., CANELLOS, G.: Cytogenetic evaluation of aneuploidy in blastic transformation of CML. Exp. Med. Intern. Cong. Series no. **233**, 187 (1971).

WHITFIELD, J. F., RIXON, R. H.: Distinctive chromosome markers of normal and radioresistant derivatives of L-strain mouse cells. Exp. Cell Res. **23**, 412 (1961).

WINGE, O.: Zytologische Untersuchungen über die Natur maligner Tumoren. I. "Crown Gall" der Zuckerrübe. Z. Zellforsch. **6**, 397 (1927).

WINGE, O.: Zytologische Untersuchungen über die Natur maligner Tumoren II. Teerkarzinome bei Mäusen. *ibid;* **10**, 683 (1930).

YAMADA, K., TAKAGI, N., SANDBERG, A. A.: Chromosomes and causation of human cancer and leukaemia. Cancer (N. Y.) **19**, 1879 (1966).

YOSHIDA, T.: Studien über des "Ascites-Sarcoma". Proc. Imp. Acad. Tokyo, **20**, 611 (1944).

YOSIDA, T. H.: Relationship between chromosomal alteration and development of tumors *in vivo* and *in vitro*. In "Cancer Cells in Culture". Tokyo: Univ. of Tokyo Press (1968).

YOSIDA, T. H., ISHIHARA, T.: Cytology of tumors. Ann. Report, Nat. Inst. Genetics (Japan) **6**, 18 (1958).

YOSIDA, T. H., OHARA, H., ROSA, R. A.: Chromosomal alteration and the development of tumors. XVII. Karyotypes of a 5-fluorodeoxyuridine resistant subline in the mouse lymphocytic neoplasma P388 growing *in vitro*. Jap. J. Genetics **43**, 49 (1968).

YOSIDA, T. H., KUROKI, T., MASUJI, H., SATO, H.: Chromosomal alteration and the development of tumors. XX. Chromosome change in the course of malignant transformation *in vitro* of hamster embryonic cells by 4-nitroquinaline 1-oxide and its derivative 4-hydroxyaminoquinoline 1-Oxide. Gann **61**, 131 (1970).

ZUR HAUSEN, H., SCHULTE-HOLTHAUSEN, H., KLEIN, G., HENLE, W., HENLE, G., CLIFFORD, P. SANTESSON, L.: EBV DNA in biopsies of Burkitt tumours and anaplastic carcinomas of the nasopharynx. Nature (Lond.) **228**, 1056 (1970).

Subject Index

Monographs already Published

In Production

In Preparation